Consultations in Liver Disease

Editor

STEVEN L. FLAMM

CLINICS IN LIVER DISEASE

www.liver.theclinics.com

Consulting Editor
NORMAN GITLIN

February 2023 • Volume 27 • Number 1

ELSEVIER

1600 John F. Kennedy Boulevard • Suite 1800 • Philadelphia, Pennsylvania, 19103-2899

http://www.theclinics.com

CLINICS IN LIVER DISEASE Volume 27, Number 1
February 2023 ISSN 1089-3261, ISBN-13: 978-0-323-96132-5

Editor: Kerry Holland
Developmental Editor: Ann Gielou M. Posedio

Clinics in Liver Disease (ISSN 1089-3261) is published quarterly by Elsevier Inc., 360 Park Avenue South, New York, NY 10010-1710. Months of issue are February, May, August, and November. Business and Editorial Offices: 1600 John F. Kennedy Blvd., Ste. 1800, Philadelphia, PA 19103-2899. Customer Service Office: 3251 Riverport Lane, Maryland Heights, MO 63043. Periodicals postage paid at New York, NY and additional mailing offices. Subscription prices are $339.00 per year (U.S. individuals), $100.00 per year (U.S. student/resident), $674.00 per year (U.S. institutions), $434.00 per year (international individuals), $200.00 per year (international student/resident), $837.00 per year (international instituitions), $393.00 per year (Canadian individuals), $100.00 per year (Canadian student/resident), and $837.00 per year (Canadian institutions). Foreign air speed delivery is included in all *Clinics* subscription prices. All prices are subject to change without notice. **POSTMASTER:** Send address changes to *Clinics in Liver Disease*, Elsevier Health Sciences Division, Subscription Customer Service, 3251 Riverport Lane, Maryland Heights, MO 63043. **Customer Service: Telephone: 1-800-654-2452 (U.S. and Canada); 314-447-8871 (outside U.S. and Canada). Fax: 314-447-8029. E-mail: journalscustomer service-usa@elsevier.com (for print support); journalsonlinesupport-usa@elsevier.com (for online support).**

Reprints. For copies of 100 or more of articles in this publication, please contact the Commercial Reprints Department, Elsevier Inc., 360 Park Avenue South, New York, NY 10010-1710. Tel.: 212-633-3874; Fax: 212-633-3820; E-mail: reprints@elsevier.com.

Clinics in Liver Disease is covered in *MEDLINE/PubMed (Index Medicus)*, Science Citation Index Expanded, Journal Citation Reports/Science Edition, and Current Contents/Clinical Medicine.

Contributors

CONSULTING EDITOR

NORMAN GITLIN, MD, FRCP (LONDON), FRCPE (EDINBURGH), FAASLD, FACP, FACG
Head of Hepatology, Southern California Liver Centers, San Clemente, California

EDITOR

STEVEN L. FLAMM, MD
Professor of Medicine, Department of Medicine, Rush University Medical School,
Department of Gastroenterology and Hepatology, Rush University Medical Center,
Chicago, Illinois

AUTHORS

JOSEPH AHN, MD
Professor of Medicine, Division of Gastroenterology and Hepatology, Oregon Health &
Science University, Portland, Oregon

ROBERT S. BROWN Jr, MD, MPH
Division of Gastroenterology and Hepatology, NewYork-Presbyterian/Weill Cornell
Medical Center, New York, New York

ADAM P. BUCKHOLZ, MD, MS
Division of Gastroenterology and Hepatology, NewYork-Presbyterian/Weill Cornell
Medical Center, New York, New York

PATRICK T. CAMPBELL, MD
Division of Gastroenterology and Hepatology, University of North Carolina School of
Medicine, Chapel Hill, North Carolina

OREN K. FIX, MD, MSc
Professor of Medicine, Division of Gastroenterology and Hepatology, University of North
Carolina School of Medicine, Chapel Hill, North Carolina

STEVEN L. FLAMM, MD
Professor of Medicine, Department of Medicine, Rush University Medical School,
Department of Gastroenterology and Hepatology, Rush University Medical Center,
Chicago, Illinois

PREVIN GANESAN, MD, MPH
Internal Medicine Resident, Northwestern University, Chicago, Illinois

DEWAN GIRI, MBBS
Department of Medicine, Mount Sinai Beth Israel, New York, New York

ROBERT G. GISH, MD
Adjunct Professor, University of California, San Diego, Skaggs School of Pharmacy and Pharmaceutical Sciences, Adjunct Professor, University of Nevada, Reno School of Medicine, Reno, Nevada

FREDRIC D. GORDON, MD
Lahey Hospital & Medical Center, Burlington, Massachusetts

JACQUELINE B. HENSON, MD
Fellow, Division of Gastroenterology, Department of Medicine, Duke University, Durham, North Carolina

PATRICK S. KAMATH, MD
Professor of Medicine, Division of Gastroenterology and Hepatology, Department of Medicine, Mayo Clinic, Rochester, Minnesota

GRES KARIM, MD
Department of Medicine, Mount Sinai Beth Israel, New York, New York

LAURA M. KULIK, MD
Professor of Medicine, Radiology, and Surgery (Organ Transplantation), Northwestern University, NMH/Arkes Family Pavilion, Chicago, Illinois

TATYANA KUSHNER, MD, MSCE
Division of Liver Diseases, Department of Obstetrics, Gynecology, and Reproductive Sciences, Icahn School of Medicine at Mount Sinai, New York, New York

PAUL Y. KWO, MD
Professor of Medicine, Director of Hepatology, Stanford University School of Medicine, Redwood City, California

YU KUANG LAI, MD
Clinical Assistant Professor, Pulmonary, Allergy and Critical Care, Department of Medicine, Stanford University, Palo Alto, California

CAROLINE L. MATCHETT, MD
Resident Physician, Internal Medicine Residency Program, Department of Medicine, Mayo Clinic, Rochester, Minnesota

ANDREW J. MUIR, MD
Professor, Department of Medicine, Division of Gastroenterology, Duke University, Duke Clinical Research Institute, Durham, North Carolina

PARITA VIRENDRA PATEL, MD
Piedmont Transplant Institute Liver Diseases and Transplantation, Atlanta, Georgia

NANCY REAU, MD
Division of Hepatology, Rush University Medical Center, Chicago, Illinois

BETHANY REUTEMANN, MD, MSc
Hepatology and Liver Transplantation, Parkland Medical Center, Derry, New Hampshire

ANN ROBINSON, MD
Gastroenterology and Hepatology Fellow, California Pacific Medical Center, San Francisco, California

RANYA SELIM, MD
Physician, Division of Gastroenterology and Hepatology, Henry Ford Health System, Detroit, Michigan

DOUGLAS A. SIMONETTO, MD
Associate Professor of Medicine, Division of Gastroenterology and Hepatology, Department of Medicine, Mayo Clinic, Rochester, Minnesota

ROBERT WONG, MD, MS
Clinical Associate Professor (Affiliated), Gastroenterology and Hepatology, Stanford University, Palo Alto, California

Contents

Evaluation of the Patient with Markedly Abnormal Liver Enzymes   1

Bethany Reutemann and Fredric D. Gordon

> Liver enzyme tests are very commonly ordered by physicians, and when
> they return as abnormal, they can pose a clinical challenge to the provider.
> Markedly abnormal liver enzymes indicate severe hepatic injury and
> require immediate evaluation. There are various causes for abnormal liver
> tests, including infectious, autoimmune, genetic, metabolic, drug, and
> vascular causes. An understanding of the patterns of aminotransferase
> and alkaline phosphatase elevations is useful in narrowing the differential
> diagnosis. A thorough history and physical examination, appropriate blood
> testing, and imaging are typically key to evaluating the patient with
> abnormal liver enzymes.

Chronic Hepatitis B Virus and Hepatitis D Virus: New Developments   17

Ann Robinson, Robert Wong, and Robert G. Gish

> Hepatitis B virus (HBV) and hepatitis D virus are leading causes of
> morbidity and mortality worldwide. Despite the availability of HBV vaccina-
> tions that are 98% to 100% effective, an estimated 820,000 annual deaths
> were attributed to HBV in 2019, mainly related to the sequelae of cirrhosis
> and hepatocellular carcinoma. Because disease prevalence is concen-
> trated outside of the United States, it is overlooked, but with expanded
> vaccination recommendations provided by the Centers for Disease Con-
> trol and Prevention and recommended screening, as well as heightened
> awareness by health care providers, we can work toward the eradication
> of this preventable disease.

Coronavirus Disease-2019 and Implications on the Liver   27

Patrick T. Campbell and Oren K. Fix

> The coronavirus disease-2019 (COVID-19) pandemic has had a large
> impact on patients with chronic liver disease (CLD) and liver transplanta-
> tion (LT) recipients. Patients with advanced CLD are at a significantly
> increased risk of poor outcomes in the setting of severe acute respiratory
> syndrome coronavirus 2 infection. The pandemic has also considerably
> altered the management and care that is provided to patients with CLD,
> pre-LT patients, and LT recipients. Vaccination against COVID-19 protects
> patients with CLD and LT recipients from adverse outcomes and is safe in
> these patients; however, vaccine efficacy may be reduced in LT recipients
> and other immunosuppressed patients.

> Pruritus can be associated with chronic liver disease, particularly cholestatic liver disease. Although the pathophysiology is uncertain, there are a few proposed mechanisms and much is still being discovered. Workup involves an assessment to rule out a dermatologic, neurologic, psychogenic, or other underlying systemic disorder. First-line therapy is cholestyramine, which is generally well tolerated and effective. In those who fail cholestyramine, alternative drugs including rifampicin and μ-opioid receptor antagonists can be considered. If medical therapy is ineffective and pruritus is significant, alternative experimental therapies such as albumin dialysis, photopheresis, plasmapheresis, and biliary diversion can be considered.

> Renal failure is one of the most prevalent complications in patients with cirrhosis and is of the utmost prognostic relevance. Acute kidney injury (AKI) in cirrhosis results from a spectrum of etiologies, of which hepatorenal syndrome (HRS) carries the worst prognosis. Correct differentiation of the etiology of AKI in cirrhosis is imperative, as treatment defers substantially. This review summarizes the current diagnostic criteria, pathophysiology, diagnosis, and therapeutic concepts for AKI and HRS–AKI in cirrhosis.

> PoPH is a well-recognized complication of portal hypertension with or without cirrhosis and is classified as a subset of PAH. Identification of PoPH is crucial as it has a major impact on prognosis and liver transplant candidacy. Echocardiogram is the initial screening tool of choice and the patient should proceed to RHC for confirmation. PAH-directed therapy is the treatment of choice, allowing the patient to achieve a hemodynamic threshold to undergo a liver transplant safely.

> This is a review of current practices and upcoming developments regarding hepatocellular carcinoma (HCC). This includes a contemporary review of the diagnosis, staging, and treatment of HCC. Furthermore, the authors provide a review of certain ongoing trials and future directions of various treatment modalities for HCC.

> Abnormal liver tests are common after liver transplantation. The differential diagnosis depends on the clinical context, particularly the time course, pattern and degree of elevation, and donor and recipient factors. The perioperative period has distinct causes compared with months and years after transplant, including ischemia-reperfusion injury, vascular thrombosis,

and primary graft nonfunction. Etiologies seen beyond the perioperative period include biliary complications, rejection, infection, recurrent disease, and non-transplant-specific causes. The evaluation begins with a liver ultrasound with Doppler as well as appropriate laboratory testing and culminates in a liver biopsy if the imaging and laboratory testing is unrevealing.

Assessment of liver fibrosis is important as the range of liver disease management has expanded, rendering biopsy both imperfect and impractical in many situations. Noninvasive tests of fibrosis leverage laboratory, imaging and elastography techniques to estimate disease extent, often with the goal of identifying advanced fibrosis. This review attempts to summarize their utility across a broad range of possible clinical scenarios while considering the central tenets of health care quality: access, quality, and cost. For each test, it also discusses the caveats whereby each test may have reduced effectiveness and how to consider each in a typical clinical setting.

Liver disease in pregnancy often requires diagnostic and therapeutic considerations that are unique to pregnancy. Liver disease in pregnancy is commonly thought of as either liver disease unique to pregnancy, chronic liver disease, or liver disease coincidental to pregnancy. This review summarizes the approach to evaluation of liver disease in pregnancy.

The prevalence of alcohol consumption, alcohol use disorder (AUD), and alcohol-related liver disease (ALD) has exponentially increased over the last several years and rates continue to increase. Significant alcohol use can cause progression from steatosis in the liver to inflammation, fibrosis, and eventually cirrhosis. Additional risk factors for the progression of ALD disease include gender, race, and genetic predisposition. As such, it is essential for clinicians to understand and implement screening tools for early diagnosis of both AUD and ALD and be aware of emerging novel treatment options.

CLINICS IN LIVER DISEASE

FORTHCOMING ISSUES

May 2023
Update on Non-Alcoholic Steatohepatitis
Zobair M. Younossi, *Editor*

August 2023
Acute-on-Chronic Liver Failure
Nikolaos T. Pyrsopoulos, *Editor*

November 2023
Hepatitis B Virus and Hepatitis D Virus
Robert G. Gish, *Editor*

RECENT ISSUES

November 2022
Primary Biliary Cholangitis
Binu V. John, *Editor*

August 2022
Pediatric Liver Disease
Philip Rosenthal, *Editor*

May 2022
The Liver and Renal Disease
David Bernstein, *Editor*

SERIES OF RELATED INTEREST

Gastroenterology Clinics of North America
https://www.gastro.theclinics.com

THE CLINICS ARE AVAILABLE ONLINE!
Access your subscription at:
www.theclinics.com

Preface

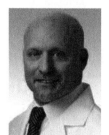

Steven L. Flamm, MD
Editor

Inpatient and outpatient consultation for patients with complex acute or chronic liver problems for Gastroenterology community practitioners is common. These encounters require detailed assessment of complicated issues and knowledge of current recommendations for optimal care. This issue of *Clinics in Liver Disease* entitled "Consultations in Liver Disease" is the fifth in a series dedicated to providing updated information to community gastroenterologists for consultations commonly encountered in practice. The first issue, entitled "Approaches to Consultation for Patients with Liver Disease," was published in 2012. The following three issues, each entitled "Consultations in Liver Disease," were published in 2015, 2017, and 2020. In each issue, concise presentations were presented that discuss clinical diagnostic and management strategies for many different liver-related problems for which practitioners are consulted. Additional topics have been selected for this issue to help community gastroenterologists care for patients with liver disease.

Markedly elevated liver enzymes are common and require urgent, targeted evaluation. Drs Reutemann and Gordon discuss diagnostic strategies. Chronic hepatitis B virus (HBV) infection and hepatitis delta virus (HDV) infection are frequently observed worldwide, but less commonly in the West. These problems are thus more complicated for the community practitioner. Drs Robinson, Wong, and Gish review the contemporary approach for diagnosis and treatment of chronic HBV and HDV.

COVID-19 has implications for liver-related disease and is a frequent reason for consultation. There is an evolving body of literature as knowledge is advanced. Dr Fix provides an updated discussion of COVID-19 and liver disease.

Pruritus is a vexing problem for patients with cholestatic liver disease, and Drs Selim and Ahn present recommendations for therapy.

Renal insufficiency and portopulmonary hypertension are two problems that portend a poor outcome for patients with liver disease, and afflicted patients are often critically ill. Drs Simonetto, Matchett, and Kamath review diagnostic and therapeutic strategies for renal insufficiency, and Dr Kwo reviews portopulmonary hypertension for the community consultant.

Clin Liver Dis 27 (2023) xi–xii
https://doi.org/10.1016/j.cld.2022.09.001
1089-3261/23/© 2022 Published by Elsevier Inc.
liver.theclinics.com

Hepatocellular carcinoma is a deadly complication for patients with advanced liver disease, and treatment approaches are rapidly evolving. Drs Ganesan and Kulik present a concise review of new developments in hepatocellular carcinoma.

Liver transplantation is a life-saving procedure for many patients with decompensated liver disease. Outcomes are optimized by careful posttransplantation care, including routine blood testing. Drs Henson and Muir discuss evaluation of an abnormal liver panel after liver transplantation.

The assessment of hepatic fibrosis is a critical aspect for patients with liver disease. In recent years, noninvasive assessment of hepatic fibrosis has played an increasingly important role in the management of such patients to avoid diagnostic liver biopsy, if possible. Drs Buckholz and Brown review strategies for noninvasive testing of hepatic fibrosis and pitfalls for which the consulting practitioner should be aware.

Liver disease in pregnancy is not uncommon and has important implications for the mother and baby. Drs Kushner and Reau review diagnostic and therapeutic recommendations in this setting.

Finally, many patients present for evaluation of alcohol-related liver disease, including alcohol-related hepatitis, and alcohol-related liver disease is a frequent reason for consultation. Dr Patel and I present current recommendations for the evaluation and management of these patients.

This issue of *Clinics in Liver Disease*, in addition to the previous issues on consultation in patients with acute and chronic liver-related problems, provides important new information for the community practitioner that will help provide appropriate care for patients with liver disease.

I would again like to thank Dr Norman Gitlin for the opportunity to serve as the editor for this issue of *Clinics in Liver Disease*. Furthermore, Kerry Holland and Ann Posedio have provided invaluable support in helping to prepare the articles for publication.

Steven L. Flamm, MD
Department of Medicine
Rush University Medical School
1725 Harrison Street, Suite 110
Chicago, IL 60612, USA

2739 Greenwood Road
Northbrook, IL 60062, USA

E-mail address:
sflamm3@outlook.com

Evaluation of the Patient with Markedly Abnormal Liver Enzymes

Bethany Reutemann, MD, MSc[a],*, Fredric D. Gordon, MD[b]

KEYWORDS

- Aminotransferase • Alkaline phosphatase • Liver enzymes • Acute liver injury
- Diagnostic algorithm • Evaluation of abnormal liver enzymes

KEY POINTS

- There is controversy surrounding the appropriate cutoff levels for aminotransferases.
- There are a multitude of causes for abnormal liver tests, including infectious, autoimmune, genetic, metabolic, drug, and vascular causes.
- An understanding of the patterns of aminotransferase and alkaline phosphatase elevations is useful in narrowing the differential diagnosis.
- The diagnostic workup of abnormal liver enzymes includes thorough history and physical examination, appropriate laboratory studies, imaging, and in some cases, liver biopsy.

INTRODUCTION

Liver chemistries are frequently ordered by health care providers during routine blood work in both the clinic and the hospital setting. When these tests, which include aspartate aminotransferase (AST), alanine aminotransferase (ALT), alkaline phosphatase (AP), and bilirubin, return abnormal, further workup is indicated in order to identify the underlying cause. Hepatocellular injury is defined as predominant elevation in AST and ALT levels, whereas cholestatic injury is defined as a predominant elevation in AP. Bilirubin, particularly conjugated bilirubin, can be elevated in either hepatocellular or cholestatic injury. Marked elevations in liver enzymes, particularly transaminases, are alarming for physicians and can indicate severe liver injury. Acute liver injury is defined as marked elevations in serum transaminases in a patient with no preexisting liver conditions in the absence of coagulopathy (international normalized ratio <1.5) and altered mental status. The authors review the background and biochemistry behind liver enzymes, provide overviews of the various conditions that can cause abnormal liver enzymes, with special focus on those conditions that can

[a] Dartmouth Hitchock Medical Center, 100 Hitchcock Way, Manchester, NH 03104, USA; [b] Tufts Medical Center, 800 Washington St. #40, South Building, 4th floor, Boston, MA 02111, USA
* Corresponding author.
E-mail address: Bethany.reutemann@gmail.com

Clin Liver Dis 27 (2023) 1–16
https://doi.org/10.1016/j.cld.2022.08.007
1089-3261/23/© 2022 Elsevier Inc. All rights reserved.

present with acute liver injury, and discuss the evaluation of the patient with abnormal liver enzymes. The workup of elevated liver enzymes following liver transplantation and during pregnancy is outside of the scope of this article and will not be covered. Management of acute liver failure is covered elsewhere in this issue.

Aminotransferases

The aminotransferases are the most frequently measured indicators of liver disease. These enzymes catalyze the reversible transfer of the amine group of aspartic acid and alanine to the α-keto group of ketoglutaric acid, which results in oxaloacetic acid (via AST), pyruvic acid (via ALT), and glutamic acid. ALT plays a key role in the intermediary metabolism of glucose and amino acids. AST is a critical enzyme regulating glutamate levels, participating in hepatic glucose synthesis during development, and in adipocyte glyceroneogenesis.[1] These reduction reactions occur in numerous organs in the body (**Table 1**)[2] and can be indicators of necrosis. In the peripheral circulation, the aminotransferases serve no metabolic function and reflect normal cell turnover. They are likely cleared by macrophage endocytosis in the liver, spleen, and bone marrow.[3,4] The half-life of ALT is approximately 50 hours, and the half-life of AST is approximately 20 hours.[5]

Serum levels of the aminotransferases are highly variable within populations and individuals. Factors affecting levels include sex, age, ethnicity, anthropomorphic features, environmental factors, diurnal variation, and heritability. The Third National Health and Nutrition Examination Survey (NHANES) study showed the prevalence of aminotransferase elevation in the general population was 9% and associated with adiposity and the metabolic syndrome.[6]

Normal laboratory values are defined as the range of values that include up to 2 standard deviations from the mean. Thus, 2.5% of a normal population will be greater than the upper limit of normal (ULN) and 2.5% of a normal population will be below. Given the numerous factors influencing the aminotransferase levels, it has been difficult to accurately ascertain a "normal range." A large study excluding patients with abnormal viral serologies and body mass index (BMI) greater than 24.9 kg/m^2 proposed that the normal ALT for women is 19 IU/L, and, for men, 30 IU/L.[7] Using the 1999 to 2002 and 2005 to 2008 NHANES databases excluding subjects with viral hepatitis, significant alcohol use, diabetes, BMI greater than 25, or enlarged waist

Table 1
Distribution of aminotransferases in human tissue expressed as a ratio to that found in human serum[2]

Tissue	AST	ALT
Liver	7000	2200
Heart	7700	350
Skeletal muscle	4800	250
Kidney	4500	950
Brain	2500	50
Pancreas	1400	100
Spleen	700	60
Lung	500	35
Erythrocytes	40	7
Serum	1	1

circumference, the maximum ULN for women was 22 IU/L and 29 IU/L for men.[8] Accumulating data have suggested that liver-related death and all-cause mortality are increased in subjects with AST or ALT elevations above these levels.[5,9–12]

The decision to decrease the accepted ULN of the AST and ALT remains controversial. Analyzing the NHANES databases, this reclassification would result in 36% of men and 28% of women meeting the new definition of abnormal liver enzymes.[13] This would likely result in increased resource utilization, unnecessary evaluations, and reduction in acceptable blood donations without a significant impact on population health. It is well-recognized that several liver diseases, including hepatitis C (HCV), hemochromatosis, and nonalcoholic fatty liver disease (NAFLD), can be significant despite normal liver enzymes. It therefore seems reasonable to increase awareness of the potential health implications of an elevated ALT $\geq$ 25 IU/L for women and $\geq$33 IU/L for men in individuals with risk factors for liver disease.[14]

Alkaline Phosphatase

AP is a group of enzymes that hydrolyze organic phosphate esters into an organic radical and inorganic phosphate. AP is present in many organs, including liver, bone, small intestine, kidney, placenta, and leukocytes. AP detected in serum is primarily sourced from liver, bone, and small intestine. Normal elevations in AP are seen in children and adolescents owing to bone growth, in late pregnancy owing to the placenta, and in people over the age of 60 years.[15–17] In pathologic states, tissues that undergo metabolic stimulation produce excess amounts of AP, which then result in elevations in serum AP. In the normal liver, AP is located on the exterior surface of the bile canalicular membrane. When bile flow is impaired, AP production is upregulated on the hepatocyte plasma membrane, which allows direct entry into the bloodstream.[18]

CAUSES OF MARKEDLY ABNORMAL LIVER ENZYMES
Viral Hepatitis

Infection with hepatitis A, B, C, delta (D), and E viruses can cause elevations in aminotransferases. Hepatitis A and E commonly cause acute hepatitis; hepatitis B and D can be acute or chronic, and HCV is typically chronic. Hepatitis B (HBV) can rarely present as acute fulminant hepatitis. Acute viral hepatitis presents with markedly abnormal aminotransferases, sometimes exceeding 1000 IU/L, whereas chronic viral hepatitis usually presents with mildly abnormal or even normal values.

Acute hepatitis A infection can be diagnosed by detection of the hepatitis A immunoglobulin M (IgM) antibody.[19] A positive hepatitis IgG antibody signifies past infection with hepatitis A or immunity. The diagnosis of HBV is usually made by the presence of hepatitis B surface antigen (HBsAg), although sometimes HBV core IgM antibody is the only clue to the diagnosis.[20] In the latter case, the diagnosis can be confirmed with an HBV DNA viral load. Chronic versus acute infection is defined by the presence of HBsAg for at least 6 months.[21] The presence of hepatitis B surface antibody (HBsAb) indicates prior vaccination or naturally occurring immunity through prior infection.[20] Hepatitis D can only replicate in a host with HBV infection. Diagnosis of hepatitis D is most reliably done through detection of hepatitis D RNA by reverse transcriptase–polymerase chain reaction.[22] HCV infection is typically screened by anti-HCV antibody testing and confirmed with HCV RNA detection.[23] Chronic HCV is defined by the presence of HCV RNA in the serum for at least 6 months. Hepatitis E is rare in the United States but is a major public health problem, particularly in Asia, the Middle East, northern Africa, and India.[24] Hepatitis E infection typically causes acute, self-limited illness and is diagnosed by anti-hepatitis E virus antibodies (IgG/IgM). HEV can cause fulminant hepatic failure most commonly seen in pregnant women.

Several other viruses, which are not primarily hepatotropic, may also cause hepatitis. These are usually herpesviruses, which can cause either chronic infections or enter a period of latency. Eight human herpesviruses have been reported to cause hepatitis: herpes simplex virus 1 and 2 (HSV1 and HSV2), varicella-zoster virus (VZV), Epstein-Barr virus (EBV), Cytomegalovirus (CMV), and human herpesviruses 6, 7, and 8. HSV hepatitis can progress to fulminant hepatitis, which presents with a characteristic pattern of liver test abnormalities, the so-called anicteric hepatitis with minimal elevations in serum bilirubin in the presence of marked elevations in the levels of serum transaminases. Early administration of high-dose intravenous acyclovir (5–10 mg/kg 3 times daily) is the key to treatment.[25] VZV hepatitis is primarily a self-limiting illness of childhood; however, clinical hepatitis in the context of disseminated VZV can be fatal, albeit rarely. Similar to HSV, VZV is best managed with high-dose acyclovir.[25] EBV hepatitis is often seen in the setting of acute infectious mononucleosis. Most cases are mild and resolve spontaneously, although acute hepatic failure in immunocompetent patients has occasionally occurred. CMV infection and CMV hepatitis are typically mild in immunocompetent patients and often resolve spontaneously; however, CMV hepatitis in immunocompromised patients, including those with AIDS and solid organ transplants, is more serious and can cause major organ damage or mortality.[26]

Autoimmune Hepatitis

Autoimmune hepatitis (AIH) is an immune-mediated chronic inflammatory disorder of the liver involving the loss of tolerance to hepatic tissue antigens. Overall, approximately 25% of patients show an acute onset of AIH, and rare cases of progression to acute or fulminant liver failure have been reported.[27] A diagnosis of AIH is based on the presence of characteristic laboratory features, including elevated aminotransferases, which can range from 2 to 40× ULN and histology, in addition to the exclusion of other hepatobiliary diseases. The presence of circulating autoantibodies (antinuclear, anti–smooth muscle, and anti–liver-kidney microsome-1) is suggestive of AIH and is further strengthened by the presence of hypergammaglobulinemia, specifically an elevated IgG, often greater than 2 g/L. The diagnosis of AIH cannot be confidently made without liver biopsy demonstrating compatible histologic findings. The hallmark histologic finding on liver biopsy is interface hepatitis, which is a predominantly periportal, lymphoplasmacytic infiltrate often accompanied by plasma cells.[28] AIH diagnosis can be facilitated by the revised AIH diagnostic scoring system developed by the International Autoimmune Hepatitis Group.[29]

Drug-Induced Liver Injury

One of the most common and potentially most deadly causes of drug-induced liver injury (DILI) is acetaminophen, which is a dose-dependent direct hepatotoxin and can cause marked elevations in serum transaminases (>1000 IU/L). Acetaminophen, one of the most frequently used pain medications available over the counter, is responsible for almost 50% of all acute liver failure cases in the United States, the United Kingdom, and many Western countries.[30] Acetaminophen is not only found in specific pain medications, but is also present in sleeping aids, medicine for colds, and numerous other over-the-counter drugs. Acetaminophen is generally a safe drug at therapeutic doses of ≤4 g per day for an adult, but an intentional or unintentional overdose can cause severe liver injury and even acute liver failure.[31] Even small to moderate use of alcohol can deplete hepatic glutathione resulting in an increased risk of acetaminophen hepatotoxicity. The only Food and Drug Administration–approved antidote against acetaminophen-induced liver injury is *N*-acetylcysteine (NAC). NAC is most effective when administered within 8 hours of the overdose and can still be beneficial even after 24 hours, although the efficacy is substantially diminished.[31,32] In contrast to idiosyncratic drug toxicity, acetaminophen-induced liver injury and liver failure have a relatively high survival rate with the use of NAC.

Idiosyncratic drug toxicity is less common than DILI from direct hepatotoxins and is dose-independent and unpredictable by definition. Moreover, the severity of injury can vary significantly with some cases presenting with only mild asymptomatic elevations in liver enzymes and others presenting with acute hepatic failure. Idiosyncratic DILI is difficult to diagnose, as it presents with varying clinical, histologic, and laboratory features depending on the drug and the host's reaction. Moreover, almost any medication or supplement can cause idiosyncratic DILI. Antibiotics are the most commonly identified drug class leading to idiosyncratic DILI, but the specific implicated agents vary considerably.[33] There has also been an increase in the number of cases attributed to herbal and dietary supplements in recent times with the most frequently implicated being body-building supplements and weight-loss products that contain green-tea extract.[34] The various clinical phenotypes and histologic features of DILI with example medications can be found in **Table 2. Box 1**

Clinical recognition will always remain challenging, as most physicians will never encounter individual reactions or observe them more often than once or twice in their professional lifetime. Given the infrequency of individual reactions, www.LiverTox.nih. gov, a free interactive database, is a helpful tool for the clinician who is suspicious of DILI or who is evaluating the patient with abnormal liver enzymes of unknown cause who may be taking one or more medications.[35]

Wilson Disease

Wilson disease is a rare genetic disorder of excess copper accumulation that results in neuropsychiatric manifestations and liver disease, and rarely, fulminant hepatic failure. The diagnosis of Wilson disease is established by a combination of clinical and biochemical findings, most notably a decrease in levels of circulating serum ceruloplasmin (<20 mg/dL) or elevated 24-hour urinary copper concentration (>100 μg/24 hours), the presence of corneal Kayser-Fleischer rings, and a hepatic copper concentration greater than 250 mg/g dry weight of liver.[36] The biochemical manifestations are variable ranging from normal transaminases and AP to markedly elevated. In mild cases of Wilson disease, treatment with metal chelating agents, if symptomatic, or zinc, if asymptomatic, is effective in stabilizing or reversing the disease.[36] In fulminant hepatic failure owing to Wilson disease or hepatic insufficiency unresponsive to medical therapy, liver transplantation is the best treatment modality.[36]

Vascular Diseases of the Liver and Ischemia

Budd-Chiari syndrome (BCS) occurs as a consequence of thrombotic occlusion of hepatic venous outflow. Occlusion may occur in hepatic venules, hepatic veins, or the inferior vena cava up to the right atrium. BCS presents with the clinical triad of abdominal pain, ascites, and hepatomegaly and can present acutely or more chronically.[37] Liver enzymes may not be strikingly abnormal if chronic but are often markedly abnormal in the acute presentation. Doppler ultrasonography is key to the diagnosis. Most causes of BCS are caused by hypercoagulable states; therefore, anticoagulation is typically the mainstay of treatment. Severe cases of BCS may require angioplasty, thrombolysis, transjugular intrahepatic portosystemic shunts, or surgical

Table 2
Clinical phenotypes of drug-induced liver injury with corresponding histologic features and drug examples[35]

Clinical Phenotype	Histologic Features	Drugs Examples
Acute fatty liver with lactic acidosis	Microvesicular hepatic steatosis ± other tissue involvement	Didanosine, fialuridine
Acute hepatic necrosis	Hepatic parenchymal collapse and necrosis	Isoniazid, aspirin, niacin
Bland cholestasis	Balloon hepatocytes with minimal inflammation	Anabolic steroids
Cholestatic hepatitis	Balloon hepatocytes with inflammation, predominance of serum alkaline phosphatase elevation	Phenytoin, amoxicillin-clavulanate
Autoimmune-like hepatitis	Plasma cells & interface hepatitis with detectable autoantibodies	Nitrofurantoin, minocycline
Immunoallergic hepatitis	Skin rash, fever, eosinophilia, cholestatic or mixed pattern of injury	Trimethoprim-sulfamethoxazole
Fibrosis/cirrhosis	Hepatic collagenization with minimal inflammation	Methotrexate, amiodarone
Nodular regeneration	Microscopic or macroscopic liver nodules	Azathioprine, oxaliplatin
Nonalcoholic fatty liver	Macrosteatosis and microsteatosis, hepatocyte ballooning, and periportal inflammation	Tamoxifen
Sinusoidal obstruction syndrome	Inflammation with obliteration of central veins	Busulfan
Vanishing bile duct syndrome	Paucity of interlobular bile ducts	Amoxicillin-clavulanate, sulfonamides

decompression with portocaval shunts.[38] Patients with decompensated cirrhosis or acute liver failure may even require liver transplantation.

Hereditary hemorrhagic telangiectasia (HHT) and veno-occlusive disease (VOD) are other rare vascular causes of liver disease. HHT is a multisystem vascular disorder causing visceral arteriovenous malformations that variably affect the liver. When there is liver involvement, it can be asymptomatic or symptomatic. Liver enzymes may be normal, or cholestasis and biliary abnormalities may occur from ischemic injury related to hepatic artery to hepatic vein shunting. More severe symptomatic cases can present with high-output heart failure, portal hypertension, or hepatic encephalopathy (HE). VOD, also known as sinusoidal obstructive syndrome, is a condition that occurs when there is obstruction of the hepatic sinusoids or small intrahepatic veins. In contrast to BCS, VOD is not thrombotic but occurs as a result of fibro-obliterative endophlebitis. It is most commonly associated with bone marrow transplantation as

---

Box 1
Noninvasive methods to predict advanced fibrosis in patients with nonalcoholic fatty liver disease[51]

Scoring systems
- NAFLD fibrosis score
- FIB-4 index
- AST to platelet ratio index (APRI)

Serum biomarkers
- Enhanced liver fibrosis (ELF) panel
- FibroTest
- Fibrosure
- Hepascore

Imaging
- Transient elastography
- Magnetic resonance elastography (MRE)
- Supersonic shear wave elastography

---

a result of certain conditioning chemotherapeutic agents used.[39] Patients often present 1 to 3 weeks after exposure with sudden-onset right upper quadrant pain, hepatomegaly, edema, and ascites.[38] Aminotransferase elevations can be marked with no or mild elevations of AP, although some cases may present with jaundice. Transjugular liver biopsy is the preferred modality for diagnosis.[38]

Ischemic hepatitis is a common cause of markedly abnormal transaminases in the critical care and postoperative settings. It occurs in the setting of acute and severe hypotension and is associated with abrupt profound elevations in liver transaminases (usually >3000 IU/L), which return to normal within several days of adequate circulatory perfusion. Often the serum bilirubin will rise as the transaminases are trending down, peaking 3 to 5 days after the peak in transaminases. Treatment is supportive.

CAUSES OF MILD TO MODERATE LIVER ENZYME ABNORMALITIES
Alcohol-Related Liver Disease

Alcohol-related liver disease (ALD) encompasses a variety of clinical disorders: steatosis, alcohol-related acute liver failure (AR-ALF, formerly known as alcoholic hepatitis), and alcohol-associated cirrhosis (AC). In the United States, ALD competes with chronic HCV as the leading indication for liver transplantation.[40] Alcohol affects the liver depending on the dose and the duration of use.[41] The most common form of ALD, alcohol-related steatosis, is likely underdiagnosed, as patients are asymptomatic. The more severe presentations of ALD, including AR-ALF and AC, present with jaundice, hepatomegaly, and portal hypertension. Although most heavy drinkers develop fatty livers, only a minority of individuals who ingest significant amounts of alcohol progress beyond fatty liver and develop AR-ALF or cirrhosis. Several risk factors have been proposed, including malnutrition, diet, gender, type of alcohol ingested, genetics, and the coexistence of viral hepatitis, but none of them individually or in combination completely explain why only a minority of those who ingest large quantities of alcohol develop ALD.

Alcohol has varying effects on the liver enzymes depending on the dose and the duration of use. Liver enzymes can range from normal to up to 10 times the ULN, and an AST/ALT ratio of greater than 2 is highly suggestive of ALD.[41,42] The peak AST or ALT in ALD is rarely greater than 400 IU/L, and higher levels suggest an alternate or additional diagnosis. In early alcohol-related steatosis, liver enzymes may be normal, or elevations may have an AST/ALT ratio of less than 2.[43,44]

ALD is often diagnosed by history and exclusion of any other potential causes of liver disease; however, biomarkers of alcohol use can be helpful in establishing or supporting the diagnosis. These biomarkers include urine ethyl glucuronide and ethyl sulfate as well as blood phosphatidylethanol.[45,46] The American Society of Addiction Medicine suggests the use of alcohol biomarkers as an aid to diagnosis, to support recovery, and as facilitators for discussion with the patient, instead of as tools to "catch" or punish patients.[47]

Nonalcoholic Fatty Liver Disease

NAFLD has become the most common cause of elevated liver enzymes, although aminotransferases are typically only mildly elevated or even normal. Components of metabolic syndrome, especially obesity and type 2 diabetes, are the most highly associated risk factors for NAFLD. The diagnosis of NAFLD requires the presence of hepatic steatosis by imaging, no significant alcohol consumption, no alternative or coexisting causes for chronic liver disease, and no other cause for the hepatic steatosis.

Nonalcoholic steatohepatitis (NASH) is a subset of NAFLD. In 1 study, the prevalence of NASH among patients with NAFLD who had a liver biopsy for a "clinical indication" was estimated to be 59%.[48] The differentiation of NAFLD from NASH is important, as patients with histologic NASH have an increased liver-related mortality rate, and it is now considered the third-most common cause of hepatocellular carcinoma in the United States.[48–50] The gold standard for the diagnosis of NASH is liver biopsy; however, it is not recommended to perform liver biopsy on every patient with NAFLD. There are several noninvasive methods to predict advanced fibrosis in patients with NAFLD, which can be found in **Box 1**.[51] Liver biopsy should be considered in patients with NAFLD who are at increased risk of having steatohepatitis and/or advanced fibrosis, when there are disparate data, or when there is concern for coexisting liver disease entities.

Cholestatic Liver Disease

Primarily intrahepatic cholestatic diseases, such as primary biliary cholangitis (PBC) and primary sclerosing cholangitis (PSC), as well as extrahepatic biliary obstruction result in increased serum AP. Transaminases may also be mildly elevated. Certain disorders, including partial biliary obstruction, tuberculosis, and other infiltrative diseases, can also cause disproportionate or isolated elevations in AP.

PBC, formerly known as primary biliary cirrhosis, is a chronic, progressive disease of unknown cause characterized by liver histology demonstrating necrosis of intrahepatic bile ducts that leads to chronic cholestasis, portal fibrosis, and cirrhosis if left untreated. PBC is more often diagnosed in women (90%), and in combination with PSC, represents the most commonly encountered causes of cholestatic liver disease, as characterized by a predominant elevation in AP rather than aminotransferases. The diagnosis of PBC should be suspected in patients with chronic cholestasis after exclusion of other causes of liver disease, particularly in middle-aged women with unexplained elevations in AP and/or persistent pruritus. The diagnosis is generally confirmed by the presence of serum antimitochondrial antibody. A liver biopsy can be used to further substantiate the diagnosis but is rarely needed unless there is concern for AIH overlap syndrome.[52]

PSC is a progressive, cholestatic liver disease that is characterized by diffuse chronic inflammation and fibrosis of the intrahepatic and extrahepatic bile ducts causing multifocal bile duct strictures.[53] The prognosis of PSC is variable, but can lead to biliary cirrhosis, which can be complicated by portal hypertension and end-stage liver disease. Although the cause of PSC remains unknown, it affects primarily young to middle-aged men and is often associated with inflammatory bowel disease, frequently ulcerative colitis.[54] Imaging of the biliary tree is essential for establishing the diagnosis of PSC. Endoscopic retrograde cholangiopancreatography (ERCP) is the gold-standard imaging modality for PSC, although clinically, magnetic resonance cholangiography (MRCP) is used more frequently, as it is more cost-effective and is almost equally sensitive and specific for the detection of PSC without exposing patients to the procedural and radiation risks of ERCP.[55] Diagnostic criteria for PSC include the following: (1) typical cholangiographic findings involving any part of the biliary tree; (2) compatible clinical and biochemical findings (ie, cholestasis for more than 6 months); (3) exclusion of causes of secondary sclerosing cholangitis (**Box 2**) and IgG4-associated cholangitis. In patients with features of cholestatic liver disease but also significantly elevated transaminases (>5× ULN), a diagnosis of AIH-PSC overlap syndrome must be considered.[56] The most feared complication of PSC is cholangiocarcinoma, which may occur in 7% to 15% of patients with PSC and does not correlate with severity of PSC.[57]

Genetic and Metabolic Disease

Hereditary hemochromatosis (HH) is one of the most common identified genetic conditions in Caucasians, especially those of northern European origin, in which it occurs with a prevalence of 1 per approximately 250 individuals.[58] The condition is typically hepatocellular in pattern, and the aminotransferases can range from normal to moderately elevated. HH constitutes several inherited disorders characterized by an increased intestinal absorption of iron with its subsequent accumulation in tissues. Most patients have a mutation in the HFE gene, in which 2 independent mutations

---

Box 2
Potential causes of secondary sclerosing cholangitis[62]

AIDS cholangiopathy

Choledocholithiasis

Cholangiocarcinoma (unless diagnosis of PSC previously established)

Diffuse intrahepatic metastases

Intra-arterial chemotherapy

Eosinophilic cholangitis

Histiocytosis X

Hepatic inflammatory pseudotumor

Ischemic cholangitis

Mast cell cholangiopathy

Recurrent pancreatitis

Portal hypertensive biliopathy

Recurrent pyogenic cholangitis

Bile duct trauma or surgery

Congenital abnormalities of biliary tree

are principally responsible for HFE-related HH. About 95% of persons with HFE-related HH are homozygous for the C282Y mutation.[59] In addition, some compound heterozygotes with single copies of both the C282Y and the H63D mutations have clinically significant iron overload.[59] The diagnosis of iron overload includes serum iron studies (elevated transferrin saturation, elevated serum ferritin levels), genetic testing, and sometimes liver biopsy to assess the hepatic iron concentration and degree of liver injury.[60] Regular phlebotomy therapy can prevent or reverse the accumulation of excess iron and reduces the risk of complications of HH, including cirrhosis and hepatocellular carcinoma.[60] When making this diagnosis, it is important to exclude secondary causes of iron overload.

Alpha-1-antitrypsin (A1AT) deficiency is another rare genetic disorder that can result in chronic liver disease. Homozygous protease inhibitor phenotype ZZ (PiZZ) A1AT deficiency is associated with chronic liver disease and hepatocellular carcinoma in adults and is a well-known cause of emphysema. In adults, A1AT typically presents with mildly abnormal transaminases but can also present as cirrhosis. The hepatic penetrance of PiZZ A1AT is approximately 10%. Serum levels of A1AT can be used for screening, although serum concentrations may increase with chronic inflammation; therefore, phenotype testing in conjunction with serum levels of A1AT is recommended.[61] Management of A1AT-associated liver disease is mostly supportive, but liver transplantation can be successful for severe hepatic impairment.

Other very rare metabolic/genetic diseases can cause elevated liver enzymes, including glycogen storage diseases, porphyrias, tyrosinemia, glycosylation disorders, disorders of lipid metabolism, urea cycle defects, cystic fibrosis, and mitochondrial liver disease; most of these usually present in childhood or adolescence.[62]

Nonhepatobiliary Causes of Elevated Liver Enzymes

Liver enzymes can be elevated from several nonhepatic conditions. A list of nonhepatic sources of elevated liver enzymes can be found in **Table 3.Box 3**

EVALUATION OF ABNORMAL LIVER ENZYMES

Evaluation of the patient with abnormal liver enzymes should be curated by a detailed history and thorough physical examination. The history should include a detailed history of present illness, inquiring into the presence of abdominal distension, edema, weight loss or gain, rashes, recent systemic illnesses, jaundice, pruritis, alterations in cognition, and changes in sleep-wake cycle. The past medical history should inquire specifically about preexisting autoimmune diseases, components of metabolic syndrome, neuropsychiatric illnesses, and history of inflammatory bowel disease, and past surgical history should identify any prior hepatobiliary surgeries. One should inquire into a family history of liver disease or cirrhosis, alcoholism, autoimmune disease, pulmonary disease, iron overload disorders, and hepatocellular cancer. A detailed review of medications should be performed, including specific inquiry about any over-the-counter medications or supplements, as well as any medications taken in the past 6 months that they are no longer taking. The social history should specifically address the patient's alcohol intake and quantity as well as any past or present illicit drug use or promiscuous sexual activity. Use of the CAGE questions to screen for excessive alcohol use is recommended (see Box 3). The review of systems should investigate the presence of sicca syndrome, arthritis, recent changes in menstrual cycle, symptoms suggestive of biliary colic, and occupational history to identify any risk of exposure to blood-borne pathogens and exposure to hepatotoxins.

Table 3 Nonhepatobiliary causes of elevated liver enzymes	
Laboratory Test	Nonhepatobiliary Causes of Elevation
Bilirubin	Gilbert syndrome Hemolysis Intra-abdominal bleeding Hematoma
AST	Rhabdomyolysis Myocardial infarction Congestive heart failure Strenuous exercise Macro-AST
ALT	Rhabdomyolysis Myocardial infarction Congestive heart failure Strenuous exercise
Alkaline phosphatase	Paget disease Hyperparathyroidism Osteomalacia Metastatic bone disease Recent fracture Paraneoplastic syndrome Intestinal injury (ie, perforation) Pregnancy

A thorough physical examination should be performed to assess for stigmata of chronic liver disease. Many abnormalities detected on physical examination usually do not develop until late in the course of liver disease. Patients with decompensated cirrhosis may present with physical examination findings of jaundice, palmar erythema, spider angiomata, telangiectasias, gynecomastia, caput medusa, splenomegaly, abdominal distension, and flank dullness to percussion, indicating ascites. Sarcopenia, or muscle wasting, is also a common finding in patients with decompensated cirrhosis. Patients with decompensated cirrhosis may also have overt HE, which presents as confusion and/or altered consciousness. Asterixis is present in overt HE and is the characteristic physical examination finding for HE. Covert HE is much more difficult to diagnose, as it has a subtle presentation; therefore, it is recommended to use psychometric or neurophysiological testing to detect. The most commonly used of these is the Stroop test, which is conveniently available as a smartphone "app."

Box 3 CAGE questions to screen for excessive alcohol intake[63]
1. Have you ever felt the need to Cut down on your drinking?
2. Have people Annoyed you by criticizing your drinking?
3. Have you ever felt Guilty about drinking?
4. Have you ever felt the need to drink first thing in the morning (Eye-opener) to steady your nerves or to get rid of a hangover?

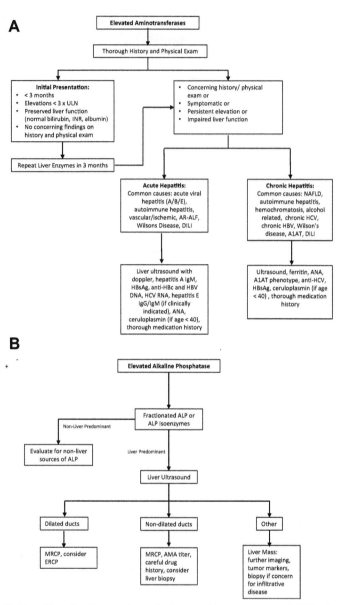

Fig. 1. (*A, B*) Algorithm for the workup of abnormal liver enzymes. A1AT, α1-antitrypsin; ALP, alkaline phosphatase; AMA, antimitochondrial antibody; ANA, antinuclear antibody; anti-HBc, anti–hepatitis B core antibody; anti-HCV, anti–hepatitis C virus; INR, international normalized ratio; MRCP, magnetic resonance cholangiography.

Based on the information gleaned from a thorough history and physical examination, specific laboratory tests can be performed for further workup. In otherwise healthy patients with previously normal liver enzymes who have liver enzyme abnormalities less than 3 times the ULN and unremarkable history and physical examination, it is reasonable to defer further workup and repeat the liver enzymes in 3 months unless their history or physical examination suggests a diagnosis. If the liver enzymes normalize, then no further workup may be necessary, and subsequent monitoring may be appropriate. If the liver enzymes remain abnormal, then further workup with additional laboratory tests and imaging is warranted. An algorithm for further workup based on the pattern of liver enzyme abnormality can be found in **Fig. 1.**

SUMMARY

Liver enzyme tests are very commonly ordered by physicians in the office during routine visits, and when they return as abnormal, they can pose a clinical challenge to the provider. Although there is still some controversy over the normal cutoffs for the tests, particularly AST and ALT, these tests are inexpensive and both sensitive and specific to screen for and monitor liver disease. There are numerous causes of abnormal liver enzymes, as reviewed in this article. A thorough history and physical examination are critically important. An understanding of the patterns of aminotransferase and AP elevations is useful in narrowing the differential diagnosis. Appropriate blood testing and imaging are required to support or confirm a diagnosis. Although liver biopsy remains a diagnostic mainstay, newer noninvasive modalities may be able to supplant a liver biopsy.

CLINICS CARE POINTS

- A true healthy normal ALT level is < 25 IU/L for women and < 33 IU/L for men in individuals with risk factors for liver disease.
- Markedly elevated liver chemistries as defined as AST and/or ALT levels > 15x the upper limit of normal and/or acute liver injury require prompt evaluation.
- There are a number of possible etiologies for abnormal liver chemistries including infectious, autoimmune, genetic, metabolic, drug, vascular, and non-hepatobiliary causes.
- Evaluation of the patient with abnormal liver chemistries includes a thorough history and physical, appropriate laboratory testing and imaging, and liver biopsy if clinicially indicated.

DISCLOSURE

No disclosures.

REFERENCES

1. Sookoian S, Pirola CJ. Liver enzymes, metabolomics and genome-wide association studies: from systems biology to the personalized medicine. World J Gastroenterol 2015;21(3):711–25.
2. Rej R. Aminotransferases in disease. Clin Lab Med 1989;9(4):667–87.
3. Horiuchi S, Kamimoto Y, Morino Y. Hepatic clearance of rate liver aspartate aminotransferase isoenzymes: evidence for endocytotic uptake via different binding sites on sinusoidal liver cells. Hepatol 1985;5(3):376–82.
4. Smit MJ, Wijnholds J, Duursma AM, et al. Plasma clearance of mitochondrial aspartate aminotransferase in the rate: competition with mitochondrial malate dehydrogenase. Biomed Biochim Acta 1986;45(11–12):1557–61.
5. Wieme RJ, Demeulenaere L. Enzyme assays in liver disease. J Clin Pathol Suppl (Assoc Clin Pathol) 1970;4:51–9.
6. Ioannou GN, Weiss NS, Boyko EJ, et al. Elevated serum alanine aminotransferase activity and calculated risk of coronary heart disease in the United States. Hepatol 2006;43:1145–51.

7. Prati D, Taioli E, Zanella A, et al. Updated definitions of healthy ranges for serum alanine aminotransferase levels. Ann Intern Med 2002;137:1–10.
8. Ruhl CE, Everhart JE. Upper limits of normal for alanine aminotransferase activity in the United States population. Hepatology 2012;55:447–54.
9. Arndt V, Brenner H, Rothenbacher D, et al. Elevated liver enzyme activity in construction workers: prevalence and impact on early retirement and all-cause mortality. Int Arch Occup Environ Health 1998;71:405–12.
10. Kim HC, Nam CM, Jee SH, et al. Normal serum aminotransferase concentration and risk of mortality from liver diseases: prospective cohort study. Br Med J 2004; 328:893.
11. Lee TH, Kim WR, Benson JT, et al. Serum aminotransferase activity and mortality risk in a United States community. Hepatol 2008;47:880–7.
12. Ruhl CE, Everhart JE. Elevated serum alanine aminotransferase and gamma-glutamyltransferase and mortality in the United States population. Gastroenterol 2009;136(477–485):e11.
13. Ioannou GN, Boyko EJ, Lee SP. The prevalence and predictors of elevated serum aminotransferase activity in the United States in 1999-2002. Am J Gastroenterol 2006;101:76–82.
14. Kwo PY, Cohen SM, Lim JK. ACG clinical guideline: evaluation of abnormal liver chemistries. Am J Gastroenterol 2017;112:18–35.
15. Clarke LC, Beck E. Plasma "alkaline phosphatase" activity. I. Normative data for growing children. J Pediatr 1950;36:335–41.
16. Birkett DJ, Done J, Neale FC, et al. Serum alkaline phosphatase in pregnancy: an immunologic study. Br Med J 1966;1:1210–2.
17. Klaassen CHL. Age and serum alkaline phosphatase. Lancet 1966;2:1361.
18. Reichling JJ, Kaplan MM. Clinical use of serum enzymes in liver disease. Dig Dis Sci 1988;12:1601–14.
19. Kao HW, Ashcavai M, Redeker AG. The persistence of hepatitis A IgM antibody after acute clinical hepatitis A. Hepatol 1984;4:933–6.
20. McMahon BJ, Alward WL, Hall DB, et al. Acute hepatitis B virus infection: relation of age to the clinical expression of disease and subsequent development of the carrier state. J Infect Dis 1985;151:599–603.
21. Terrault NA, Bzowej NH, Chang KM, et al. American Association for the Study of Liver Diseases: AASLD guidelines for treatment of chronic hepatitis B. Hepatology 2016;63:261–83.
22. Zignego AL, Deny P, Feray C, et al. Amplification of hepatitis delta virus RNA sequences by polymerase chain reaction: a tool for viral detection and cloning. Mol Cell Probes 1990;4:43–51.
23. Centers for Disease Control and Prevention. Testing for HCV infection: an update of guidance for clinicians and laboratorians. MMWR Morb Mortal Wkly Rep 2013; 62:362–5.
24. Krawczynski K, Kamili S, Aggarwal R. Global epidemiology and medical aspects of hepatitis. E. Forum (Genova) 2001;11(2):166–79.
25. Hewlett G, Hallenberger S, Rubsamen-Waigmann H. Antivirals against DNA viruses (hepatitis B and the herpes viruses). Curr Opin Pharmacol 2004;4(5): 453–64.
26. Rosen HR, Chou S, Corless CL, et al. Cytomegalovirus viremia: risk factor for allograft cirrhosis after liver transplantation for hepatitis C. Transplantation 1997; 64(5):721–6.
27. Nikias GA, Batts KP, Czaja AJ. The nature and prognostic implications of autoimmune hepatitis with acute presentation. J Hepatol 1994;19:225–32.

28. Czaja AJ, Carpenter HA. Sensitivity, specificity, and predictability of biopsy interpretations in chronic hepatitis. Gastroenterol 1993;105:1824–32.
29. Hennes EM, Zeniya M, Czaja AJ, et al. Simplified criteria for the diagnosis of autoimmune hepatitis. Hepatology 2008;48:169–76.
30. Lee WM. Acute liver failure. Semin Respir Crit Care Med 2012;33:36–45.
31. Larson AM. Acetaminophen hepatotoxicity. Clin Liver Dis 2007;11:525–48.
32. Smilkstein MJ, Knapp GL, Kulig KW, et al. Efficacy of oral N-acetylcysteine in the treatment of acetaminophen overdose. N Engl J Med 1988;319:1557–62.
33. Chalasani N, Fontana RJ, Bonkovsky HL, et al. Causes, clinical features, and outcomes from a prospective study of drug induced liver injury in the United States. Gastroenterol 2008;135:1924–34.
34. Navarro VJ, Khan I, Bjornsson E, et al. Liver injury from herbal and dietary supplements. Hepatology 2017;65:363–73.
35. LiverTox: clinical and research information on drug-induced liver injury [internet]. National Center for Biotechnology Information. Available at: https://pubmed.ncbi. nlm.nih.gov/31643176/. Accessed May 4, 2022.
36. Roberts EA, Schilsky ML. Diagnosis and treatment of Wilson disease: an update. Hepatology 2008;47:2089–111.
37. Budd G. On diseases of the liver. London: John Churchill; 1845. p. 146.
38. Northup PG, Garcia-Pagan JC, Garcia-Tsao G, et al. Vascular liver disorders, portal vein thrombosis, and procedural bleeding in patients with liver disease: 2020 practice guidance by the American association for the study of liver diseases. Hepatology 2021;73(1):366–413.
39. Jones RJ, Lee KSK, Beschorner WE, et al. Venoocclusive disease of the liver following bone marrow transplantation. Transplantation 1987;44:778–83.
40. Mellinger JL, Shedden K, Winder GS, et al. The high burden of alcoholic cirrhosis in privately insured persons in the United States. Hepatology 2018;68(3):872–82.
41. Lieber CS. Alcoholic liver disease: new insights in pathogenesis lead to new treatments. J Hepatol 2000;32(1 Suppl):113–28.
42. Ellis G, Goldberg DM, Spooner RJ, et al. Serum enzyme tests in diseases of the liver and biliary tree. Am J Clin Pathol 1978;70:248–58.
43. Cohen JA, Kaplan MM. The SGOT/SGPT ratio—an indicator of alcoholic liver disease. Dig Dis Sci 1979;24:835–8.
44. Nyblom H, Berggren U, Balldin J, et al. High AST/ALT ratio may indicate advanced alcoholic liver disease rather than heavy drinking. Alcohol Alcohol 2004;39:336–9.
45. Stewart SH, Koch DG, Burgess DM, et al. Sensitivity and specificity of urinary ethyl glucuronide and ethyl sulfate in liver disease patients. Alcohol Clin Exp Res 2013;37:150–5.
46. Schröck A, Wurst FM, Thon N, et al. Assessing phosphatidylethanol (PEth) levels reflecting different drinking habits in comparison to the alcohol use disorders identification test - C (AUDIT-C). Drug Alcohol Depend 2017;178:80–6.
47. Jarvis M, Williams J, Hurford M, et al. Appropriate use of drug testing in clinical addiction medicine. J Addict Med 2017;11:163–73.
48. Sayiner M, Koenig A, Henry L, et al. Epidemiology of nonalcoholic fatty liver disease and nonalcoholic steatohepatitis in the United States and the rest of the world. Clin Liver Dis 2016;20:205–14.
49. GBD 2015 Mortality and Causes of Death Collaborators. Global, regional, and national life expectancy, all-cause mortality, and cause-specific mortality for 249 causes of death, 1980- 2015: a systematic analysis for the Global Burden of Disease Study 2015. Lancet 2016;388:1459–544.

50. Mohamad B, Shah V, Onyshchenko M, et al. Characterization of hepatocellular carcinoma (HCC) in non-alcoholic fatty liver disease (NAFLD) patients without cirrhosis. Hepatol Int 2016;10:632–9.
51. Kaswala DH, Lai M, Afdhal NH. Fibrosis assessment in nonalcoholic fatty liver disease (NAFLD) in 2016. Dig Dis Sci 2016;61:1356–64.
52. Zein CO, Angulo P, Lindor KD. When is liver biopsy needed in the diagnosis of primary biliary cirrhosis? Clin Gastroenterol Hepatol 2003;1:89–95.
53. Maggs JR, Chapman RW. An update on primary sclerosing cholangitis. Curr Opin Gastroenterol 2008;24:377–83.
54. Fausa O, Schrumpf E, Elgjo K. Relationship of inflammatory bowel disease and primary sclerosing cholangitis. Semin Liver Dis 1991;11:31–9.
55. Soto JA, Barish MA, Yucel EK, et al. Magnetic resonance cholangiography: comparison with endoscopic retrograde cholangiopancreatography. Gastroenterol 1996;110:589–97.
56. Czaja AJ. The variant forms of autoimmune hepatitis. Ann Intern Med 1996;125:588–98.
57. Kornfield D, Ekbom A, Ihre T. Survival and risk of cholangiocarcinoma complicating primary sclerosing cholangitis: the Mayo Clinic experience. Am J Gastroenerol 2001;96:1164–9.
58. Phatak PD, Bonkovsky HL, Kowdley KV. Hereditary hemochromatosis: time for targeted screening. Ann Intern Med 2008;149:270–2.
59. Beutler E, Gelbart T, West C, et al. Mutation analysis in hereditary hemochromatosis. Blood Cells Mol Dis 1996;22:187–94.
60. Bacon BR, Adams PC, Kowdley KV, et al. Diagnosis and management of hemochromatosis: 2011 practice guideline by the American association for the study of liver diseases. Hepatology 2011;54:328–43.
61. Steiner SJ, Gupta SK, Croffie JM, et al. Serum levels of α1-antitrypsin predict phenotypic expression of the α1-antitrypsin gene. Dig Dis Sci 2003;48:1793–6.
62. Schiff ER, Sorrell MF, Maddrey WC. Schiff's disease of the liver. 10th edition. Philadelphia, PA: Lippincott Williams & Wilkins; 2007.
63. Ewing JA. Detecting alcoholism: the CAGE questionnaire. JAMA Int Med 1984;252:1905–7.

Chronic Hepatitis B Virus and Hepatitis D Virus

New Developments

Ann Robinson, MD[a], Robert Wong, MD, MS[b],
Robert G. Gish, MD[c,d],*

KEYWORDS

- Hepatitis B • Hepatitis D • Hepatitis delta • Vaccination • Antivirals

KEY POINTS

- Hepatitis B remains a leading cause of liver-related morbidity and mortality globally, and increased efforts are needed to improved screening and linkage to care.
- The Centers for Disease Control and Prevention recommends universal adult hepatitis B vaccination for infants through adults 59 years of age, which could increase vaccination coverage and decrease overall hepatitis B cases.
- Existing therapies for hepatitis B are highly effective at suppressing viral replication, and novel therapies with greater potential for functional cure are on the horizon.
- Hepatitis delta infection occurring in the setting of chronic hepatitis B is associated with the most severe form of viral hepatitis, leading to a significantly greater risk of cirrhosis, hepatocellular carcinoma, and death.
- There are currently no Food and Drug Administration-approved therapies for hepatitis delta in the United States, but novel therapies effective at suppressing hepatitis delta virus RNA are soon to become available, pending results of ongoing phase 3 clinical trials.

EPIDEMIOLOGY OF HEPATITIS B VIRUS

The prevalence of hepatitis B virus (HBV) is underestimated in many regions, due to lack of epidemiologic data from many regions where its prevalence is highest. It is estimated that 272 million people were living with chronic hepatitis B (CHB) infection in 2020, with 1.5 million new infections each year.[1,2] The highest prevalence of the

[a] California Pacific Medical Center, 1101 Van Ness Avenue, San Francisco, CA 94109, USA;
[b] Gastroenterology and Hepatology, Stanford University, 3801 Miranda Avenue, GI-111, Palo Alto, CA 94304, USA; [c] University of California San Diego, Skaggs School of Pharmacy and Pharmaceutical Sciences; [d] University of Nevada, Reno School of Medicine
* Corresponding author. Robert G. Gish Consultants, LLC, 6022 La Jolla Mesa Drive, San Diego, CA 92037.
E-mail address: rgish@robertgish.com

Clin Liver Dis 27 (2023) 17–25
https://doi.org/10.1016/j.cld.2022.08.001
1089-3261/23/© 2022 Elsevier Inc. All rights reserved.

disease is noted to be in the Western Pacific (116 million), Africa (81 million), Eastern Mediterranean (18 million), and South East Asia (16 million).[1,3]

In the United States, it was estimated that only 850,000 persons were living with HBV infection based on survey data.[4,5] However, when considering foreign-born populations and changing immigration patterns, one recent study estimates the prevalence of CHB infection to be as high as 2.4 million in the United States.[6] In addition, the incidence of acute HBV infection is increasing as noted in a study reporting an increase of 114% in three states (Kentucky, Tennessee, and West Virginia) from 2009 to 2013; this increase is thought to be related to an increase in injection drug use.[7]

VACCINATION FOR HEPATITIS B VIRUS

As of 2021, the US Centers for Disease Control and Prevention (CDC) Advisory Committee on Immunization Practices (ACIP) recommendation expands the indicated age range for universal HBV vaccination to now include all adults aged 19 to 59 years.[8] This removes the previous recommendation for risk factor assessment in this age group to determine vaccine eligibility. In addition, it is now recommended that universal vaccination be provided to those 60 years and older if they have increased risk factors for HBV, including being men who have sex with men, those having sex partners who are positive for hepatitis B surface antigen (HBsAg), those having more than 1 sex partner in 6 months, persons at risk for percutaneous or mucosal exposure to blood, those who travel to countries with high or intermediate endemic HBV ($\geq$2% HBsAg seroprevalence), persons with hepatitis C virus (HCV) or human immunodeficiency virus (HIV), those with chronic liver disease, or those who are incarcerated, as well as anyone who wishes to be vaccinated against HBV.[8] In addition, the new recommendations state that health care providers should offer HBV vaccination to all adults, including those 60 years and older, even without known risk factors, which differs from prior language suggesting that vaccination should be provided when requested by the patient. This shifts the responsibility of initiating the consideration of HBV vaccination from the patient to the provider.[8]

The World Health Organization (WHO) recommends that all infants receive the HBV vaccine as soon as possible after birth, preferably within 24 hours.[1] The vaccination is typically given as three doses administered at 0, 1, and 6 months as in the single-antigen vaccinations available with Recombivax and Energix-B or the combination hepatitis A and B vaccination, Twinrix. In addition, Twinrix may be administered on an accelerated schedule before travel, potential exposure, or immunosuppression at 0, 7, and 21 to 30 days, followed by a dose at 12 months.[4] Heplisav-B is a two-series vaccination for HBV administered at 0 and 1 months, approved for adults 18 years and older. Heplisav-B was approved by the Food and Drug Administration (FDA) in 2017; when compared with Energix-B, there was no difference in the occurrence of serious adverse events.[9] In addition, PreHevbrio is the first 3-antigen-containing vaccine, which is also a three-series vaccination, approved for HBV.[10] PreHevbrio was approved by FDA in 2021 and there is little or no difference in seroprotection or occurrence of mild or serious adverse events when compared with Engerix-B.[8]

The presence of anti-HBs $\geq$10 IU/L 1 to 2 months after three doses of vaccine is considered to be reflective of immunity. Literature suggests that the protection against HBV from full vaccination is at least 30 years and potentially lifelong due to the persistence of immunologic memory even if anti-HBs is negative.[4,11] Persons who have completed an HBV vaccination series at any point or who have a history of HBV infection should not receive additional HBV vaccination, although there is no evidence that receiving additional vaccine doses is harmful.[12] In addition, the CDC notes that there are cases where revaccination might be indicated, as in nonresponder infants born to persons testing positive for HBsAg, health care providers, and persons receiving hemodialysis.[4,8] The CDC also recommends that health care providers only accept dated records as evidence of HBV vaccination.[8]

Screening/Testing Before Vaccination

Testing is not a requirement for vaccination, and in settings where testing is not feasible, vaccination of persons recommended to receive the vaccine should continue.[4,8] However, in settings in which the patient population has a high rate of previous HBV infection, pre-vaccination testing should be performed concomitantly with the administration of the first dose of vaccine. This may reduce costs by avoiding the complete vaccination of persons who are already immune.[8] It may also reduce the risk of providing false reassurance of vaccine-induced protection in patients who have undiagnosed CHB or past exposure to HBV, as evidenced by the presence of hepatitis B core antibody (anti-HBc) total.

Serologic markers for HBV infection include HBsAg, antibody to HBsAg (anti-HBs), hepatitis B core antibody (anti-HBc), immunoglobulin M and immunoglobulin G (IgM anti-HBc, IgG anti-HBc).[4] At least 1 serologic marker is present during the different phases of acute and chronic HBV infection. The CDC recommends screening all pregnant women for HBV with HBsAg. In addition, they recommend universal screening at least once in a lifetime for all persons 18 years and older with the following 3-panel test: HBsAg, anti-HBs, and anti-HBc.[13] This replaces prior risk factor-based screening and will help differentiate persons who have a current HBV infection from those who have immunity from a prior infection but may be susceptible to reactivation, and those who are susceptible and need vaccination.[4] The Proposed Updated Recommendations from the CDC also expand existing risk-based testing recommendations to include the following populations, activities, exposures, or conditions associated with increased risk for HBV infection: persons currently or formerly incarcerated in a jail, prison, or other detention setting; persons with a history of sexually transmitted infections or multiple sex partners; and persons with a history of HCV infection.[13]

TREATMENT GUIDELINES FOR CHRONIC HEPATITIS B

The goal of CHB treatment is to prevent liver-related morbidity and mortality.[14,15] Guidelines for the treatment vary by organization, whether following the 2018 Updates on the Treatment of Hepatitis B from the American Association for the Study of Liver Diseases (AASLD), the 2017 Clinical Practice Guidelines from the European Association for the Study of the Liver (EASL), or the 2015 Update of the Asia Pacific Clinical Practice Guidelines from the Asian Pacific Association for the Study of the Liver (APASL). When deciding on timing of the initiation of therapy, it is also important to consider additional risk factors for hepatocellular carcinoma (HCC) and cirrhosis, such as the patient's age and their family history of HCC. Below are the indications for treatment in those patients who have CHB (sorted by recommending society).

American Association for the Study of Liver Diseases

The AASLD recommends treating HBV infection with antiviral therapy in patients with compensated cirrhosis if HBV DNA greater than 2000 IU/mL regardless of the alanine aminotransferase (ALT) level, and treating patients with decompensated cirrhosis with any detectable HBV DNA.[14] For CHB with HBeAg positivity, the AASLD recommends that if the ALT is lower than the upper limit of normal (<35 IU/L for men and <25 IU/L for women), and HBV DNA ≥20,000 IU/mL, the ALT and HBV DNA of these patients can be monitored every 3 to 6 months.[16] If there is a rise in ALT, but less than 2 times the upper limit of normal, with a falling HBV DNA level, this may signify seroconversion, so monitoring should be increased in frequency. Lastly, if these patients have an elevated ALT greater than 2 times the upper limit of normal, with HBV DNA ≥20,000 IU/mL, then they should be treated. For CHB with negative HBeAg activity and ALT lower than the upper limit of normal, the ALT and HBV DNA of these patients can be monitored every 3 to 6 months. If ALT increases but is less than 2 times the upper limit of normal with HBV DNA less than 2000 IU/mL, then ALT and HBV DNA can be monitored every 3 months for a year, then every 6 months. If ALT is greater than 2 times the upper limit of normal with HBV DNA ≥2000 IU/mL, then patients should be treated. The AASLD also recommends considering factors like age (>40 years), a family history of cirrhosis or HCC, previous treatment history, presence of cirrhosis, or presence of extrahepatic manifestations when deciding whether to treat patients with CHB with ALT less than two times the upper limit of normal and HBV DNA ≤2000 IU/mL in HBeAg-negative patients or ≤20,000 IU/mL in HBeAg-positive patients.

European Association for the Study of the Liver

EASL recommends that all patients with CHB who are HBeAg-positive or -negative with HBV DNA ≥2000 IU/mL, ALT at the upper limit of normal (normal is approximately 40 IU/L for men and women), or at least moderate liver necroinflammation or fibrosis be treated.[15] If patients have a normal ALT but high HBV DNA levels, they may be treated if they are older than 30 years, regardless of the severity of liver histologic lesions. Patients with both compensated and decompensated cirrhosis need treatment. Lastly, patients that have a family history of HCC or cirrhosis, and extrahepatic manifestations can be treated even if the above treatment indications are not fulfilled.[15]

Asian Pacific Association for the Study of the Liver

APASL recommends treating everyone with compensated or decompensated cirrhosis.[17] For non-cirrhotic HBeAg-positive CHB, with ALT less than 2 times the upper limit of normal (normal ≤40 IU/L for men and women) and HBV DNA less than 20,000 IU/mL, patients may be monitored every 3 months. If testing reveals moderate to severe inflammation or significant fibrosis, then treat. If ALT is ≥2 times the upper limit of normal and HBV DNA is >20,000 IU/mL without seroconversion for 3 months, then these patients should be treated. For non-cirrhotic HBeAg-negative CHB, these patients can be monitored unless ALT is 2 times the upper limit of normal with HBV DNA greater than 2000 IU/mL, in which case therapy should be initiated.

Antiviral medications can suppress HBV replication, decrease liver injury, and prevent transmission to susceptible persons.[18] Despite this, WHO estimates that only 16.7% of those diagnosed with CHB are receiving treatment.[19] In addition, some experts argue that treatment guidelines should be expanded, citing rising evidence that high viremia and persistent presence of HBeAg are associated with increased risk of cirrhosis, HCC, and liver-related mortality.[18,20–22] One US study of 41 HBeAg-positive patients with ALT ≤40 IU/L found that despite having normal ALT, many patients in the immune-tolerant phase have significant disease on liver biopsy (fibrosis stage ≥2 or fibrosis stage 1 plus grade ≥2 inflammation); this was noted in 29% of all patients, in 0% of those 35 years or younger, in 22% of those aged 36 to 50, and in 45% of those older than 50 years.[23] Overall, they report that there is data to support expanding treatment to immune tolerant and those in the indeterminate phenotype (commonly HBeAg-negative with HBV DNA <10,000 IU/mL but ALT greater than the upper limit of normal) who have evidence of active or advanced liver disease as well as treatment to immune tolerant patients older than 40 years and even possibly those older than 30 years.

PREFERRED THERAPIES FOR HEPATITIS B VIRUS

The 2018 AASLD Updates on Hepatitis B reports the preferred therapies for HBV include entecavir, tenofovir dipovoxil fumarate (TDF), tenofovir alafenamide (TAF), and pegylated -interferon (PEG-IFN).[16] Entecavir, TDF, and TAF are nucleoside/nucleotide analogs, which can be administered orally.[15] They are long-term treatments, until HBsAg loss, with early stopping considered in select cases. They are tolerated well and have good viral suppression, with minimal to no risk of viral resistance.[15] For entecavir and TDF, there are dosage adjustments based on renal function. TAF is more stable than TDF in plasma and delivers the active metabolite to hepatocytes more efficiently, allowing a lower dose to be used with similar antiviral activity, less systemic exposure, and decreased renal and bone toxicity.[16] PEG-IFN is given as subcutaneous injections for 48 weeks.[15] It is less well tolerated and has more adverse effects, namely in those with psychiatric, neurologic, and endocrine dysfunction. It provides moderate viral suppression and no risk of viral resistance.[15]

When comparing entecavir and TDF, prior studies have shown that TDF was superior to entecavir in suppressing HBV viral load while having a similar safety profile to TDF.[24] In addition, a 2019 meta-analysis comparing tenofovir monotherapy with entecavir monotherapy in patients with CHB found that the incidence of HCC was significantly lower in the tenofovir group than the entecavir group (rate ratio [95% CI] of 0.66 [0.49, 0.89]; $P = .008$), while there was no statistical significance in incidence of death or transplantation (rate ratio [95% CI] of 0.78 [0.55, 1.13]; $P = .19$), encephalopathy (risk ratio [95% CI] of 0.72 [0.45, 1.13];, $P = .15$) or variceal bleeding (risk ratio [95% CI] of 0.71 [0.34, 1.50], $P = .37$) between the 2 groups.[25]

NEW HEPATITIS B VIRUS THERAPIES ON THE HORIZON

The therapeutic goals of current antivirals are mainly virologic and biochemical responses that may prevent disease progression and improve survival; however, these therapies do not generally promise a functional cure, or sustained loss of HBsAg.[26,27] Future therapies for HBV cure include agents that target the virus life cycle or those that indirectly modulate host factor/host immune responses including entry inhibitors; core protein allosteric modulators; those that cause RNA interference, inhibition, or neutralization of HBsAg; inhibitors of cccDNA; toll-like receptor agonists; immune checkpoint inhibitors; and therapeutic vaccines.[27] While none of these novel therapies are currently available, several agents undergoing clinical trials look promising and the field continues to anxiously await interim data readouts on the efficacy of these potential agents.

COINFECTION AND SUPERINFECTION WITH HEPATITIS D

Hepatitis D, also known as "delta hepatitis," is a liver infection caused by the hepatitis D virus (HDV) and only occurs in people who are also infected with the HBV.[28] People can become infected with both hepatitis B and hepatitis D viruses at the same time, referred to as "coinfection," or get hepatitis D after first being infected with HBV, known as "superinfection."[28] Once chronicity is established, HDV can rapidly progress to cirrhosis in 10% to 15% of patients within 2 years and in 70% to 80% of patients within 5 to 10 years.[29,30]

Several recent studies have attempted to provide updated estimates of global HDV prevalence but have been limited by lack of high-quality population-level data. HDV prevalence estimates have ranged from 15 million to 72 million, although most experts believe the prevalence is likely closer to 20 million affected globally.[31–34] Like HBV, these variations in prevalence estimates likely stem from incomplete population testing due to less clinical awareness, but also may reflect a lack of availability of HDV testing.[35] Hepatitis D is most common in Eastern Europe, Southern Europe, the Mediterranean region, the Middle East, West and Central Africa, East Asia, and the Amazon Basin in South America.[28] In the United States, prevalence data for HDV is lacking, with prior studies citing a range from 2% to 50%.[35–37] In one study of 1191 patients with CHB, 499 had been tested for HDV, and 42 (8%) were determined to be coinfected; half of these were also HCV-infected. Cirrhosis was present in 73% of the coinfected, 80% of the tri-infected, but only 22% of the mono-infected. Twenty-nine patients (69%) were Caucasian/non-Hispanic; 10 (24%) were Asians and Pacific Islanders.[37] In addition, another study showed that the seroprevalence of HDV was increasing from 29% in 1988 to 1989 to 50% in 2005 to 2006 in one US city among people who inject drugs.[35,38]

The AASLD recommends testing of HBsAg-positive persons at risk for HDV, including those with HIV infection, persons who inject drugs, men who have sex with men, those at risk for sexually transmitted disease, and immigrants from areas of high HDV endemicity.[14] However, given the severity of disease caused by HDV, as well as more recent prevalence data suggesting a higher-than-expected prevalence, some experts recommend universal testing for HDV in anyone with CHB.[37,39,40] The recommended screening test for HDV is serum anti-HDV IgG followed by HDV RNA PCR if positive.[35]

The goal of HDV treatment is HDV RNA clearance or suppression with the ultimate goal of reducing progression to cirrhosis, hepatic decompensation, and HCC.[39] For persons with HDV infection, the only effective treatment currently available in the United States is pegylated-interferon-α (PEG-α).[14] In patients with active hepatitis D with elevated liver enzymes, histologic evidence of hepatitis, or persistently elevated HDV RNA or anti-HDV IgM who do not have contraindications to PEG-α, PEG-α treatment can be initiated.[39] However, the rate of sustained HDV RNA suppression after 1 year of PEG-α therapy is only 15% to 20%, and this is not a well-tolerated drug.[41,42]

Owing to the current limitations of interferon-α-based therapies, there has been interest in novel therapies for HDV.[35] Current investigational therapies target various stages of the HDV lifestyle, and include the following classes: interferon-lambda (IFN-λ), prenylation inhibitors (lonafarnib), entry inhibitors (hepcludex B), and nucleic acid polymers.[35]

CLINICS CARE POINTS

- The prevalence of hepatitis B and D are underestimated in many regions of the world, including the United States.
- The US Centers for Disease Control and Prevention (CDC) has expanded the indicated age range for universal hepatitis B virus (HBV) vaccination to now include all adults aged 19 to 59 years.
- Although antiviral medications can suppress HBV replication, decrease liver injury, and prevent transmission to susceptible persons, few with chronic hepatitis B (CHB) are receiving therapy.
- Given the severity of disease caused by hepatitis D virus (HDV), as well as a higher-than-expected prevalence, some experts recommend universal testing for HDV in anyone with CHB.

- While current therapies do not generally promise a functional cure, future therapies for HBV cure include agents that target the virus life cycle or those that indirectly modulate host factor/host immune responses.

DISCLOSURE

A. Robinson: This author has nothing to disclose. R. Wong: research funding (to his institution) from Gilead Sciences, United States; he has served as a consultant and on advisory board for Gilead Sciences. R.G. Gish: He has served as a consultant and/or advisor for Gilead Sciences.

REFERENCES

1. World Health Organization. Hepatitis B. World Health Organization; 2021. https://www.who.int/news-room/fact-sheets/detail/hepatitis-b. [Accessed 12 April 2022].
2. CDA Foundation Polaris Observatory. Prevalence of HBsAg. https://cdafound.org/premium-dashboard/. [Accessed 26 April 2022].
3. Gomes C, Wong RJ, Gish RG. Global perspective on hepatitis B virus infections in the era of effective vaccines. Clin Liver Dis 2019;23(3):383–99.
4. Schillie S, Vellozzi C, Reingold A, et al. Prevention of hepatitis B virus infection in the United States: recommendations of the Advisory Committee on Immunization Practices. MMWR Recomm Rep 2018;67(1):1–31.
5. Roberts H, Kruszon-Moran D, Ly KN, et al. Prevalence of chronic hepatitis B virus (HBV) infection in U.S. Households: National Health and Nutrition Examination survey (NHANES), 1988-2012. Hepatology 2016;63(2):388–97.
6. Wong RJ, Brosgart CL, Welch S, et al. An updated assessment of chronic hepatitis B prevalence among foreign-born persons living in the United States. Hepatology (Baltimore, Md) 2021;74(2):607–26.
7. Harris AM, Iqbal K, Schillie S, et al. Increases in acute hepatitis B virus infections - Kentucky, Tennessee, and West Virginia, 2006-2013. MMWR Morb Mortal Wkly Rep 2016;65(3):47–50.
8. Weng MK. PreHevbrio for adult hepatitis B vaccination: evidence to recommendation and GRADE. Presented February 23, 2022. https://www.cdc.gov/vaccines/acip/meetings/downloads/slides-2022-02-23-24/02-HepWG-weng-508.pdf. [Accessed 12 April 2022].
9. Schillie S, Harris A, Link-Gelles R, et al. Recommendations of the Advisory Committee on Immunization Practices for use of a hepatitis B vaccine with a novel adjuvant. MMWR Morb Mortal Wkly Rep 2018;67(15):455–8.
10. Weng MK. PreHevbrio for adult hepatitis B vaccination evidence to recommendation and GRADE. https://www.cdc.gov/vaccines/acip/meetings/downloads/slides-2022-02-23-24/02-HepWG-weng-508.pdf2022. [Accessed 12 April 2022].
11. World Health Organization. Global Health Sector Strategy on Viral Hepatitis 2016-2021. Updated May 17, 2016. https://www.who.int/publications/i/item/WHO-HIV-2016.06. [Accessed 12 April 2022].
12. Kroger A, Bahta L, Hunter P. General Best Practice Guidelines for Immunization. https://www.cdc.gov/vaccines/hcp/acip-recs/general-recs/index.html. [Accessed 12 April 2022].
13.. Centers for Disease Control and Prevention. Federal Register Notice for Hepatitis B Screening and Testing. CDC-2022-07050. https://www.cdc.gov/hepatitis/policy/isireview/HepBFederalRegisterNotice.htm2022. p. 19516-19617. [Accessed 12 April 2022].

14. Terrault NA, Bzowej NH, Chang KM, et al. AASLD guidelines for treatment of chronic hepatitis B. Hepatology 2016;63(1):261–83.
15. EASL 2017 Clinical Practice Guidelines on the Management of Hepatitis B Virus Infection. J Hepatol 2017;67(2):370–98. https://doi.org/10.1016/j.jhep.2017.03.021.
16. Terrault NA, Lok ASF, McMahon BJ, et al. Update on prevention, diagnosis, and treatment of chronic hepatitis B: AASLD 2018 Hepatitis B Guidance. Hepatology (Baltimore, Md) 2018;67(4):1560–99.
17. Sarin SK, Kumar M, Lau GK, et al. Asian-Pacific Clinical Practice Guidelines on the Management of Hepatitis B: a 2015 update. Hepatol Int 2016;10(1):1–98.
18. Jeng WJ, Lok AS. Should treatment indications for chronic hepatitis B be expanded? Clin Gastroenterol Hepatol 2021;19(10):2006–14.
19. Hutin Y, Nasrullah M, Easterbrook P, et al. Access to treatment for hepatitis B virus infection - worldwide, 2016. MMWR Morb Mortal Wkly Rep 2018;67(28):773–7.
20. Chen YC, Chu CM, Liaw YF. Age-specific prognosis following spontaneous hepatitis B e antigen seroconversion in chronic hepatitis B. Hepatology (Baltimore, Md) 2010;51(2):435–44.
21. Chen CF, Lee WC, Yang HI, et al. Changes in serum levels of HBV DNA and alanine aminotransferase determine risk for hepatocellular carcinoma. Gastroenterology 2011;141(4):1240–8, 1248.e1-2.
22. McNaughton AL, Lemoine M, van Rensburg C, et al. Extending treatment eligibility for chronic hepatitis B virus infection. Nat Rev Gastroenterol Hepatol 2021;18(3):146–7.
23. Nguyen MH, Garcia RT, Trinh HN, et al. Histological disease in Asian-Americans with chronic hepatitis B, high hepatitis B virus DNA, and normal alanine aminotransferase levels. Am J Gastroenterol 2009;104(9):2206–13.
24. Zuo SR, Zuo XC, Wang CJ, et al. A meta-analysis comparing the efficacy of entecavir and tenofovir for the treatment of chronic hepatitis B infection. J Clin Pharmacol 2015;55(3):288–97.
25. Zhang Z, Zhou Y, Yang J, et al. The effectiveness of TDF versus ETV on incidence of HCC in CHB patients: a meta analysis. BMC Cancer 2019;19(1):511.
26. Naggie S, Lok AS. New therapeutics for hepatitis B: the road to cure. Annu Rev Med 2021;72:93–105.
27. Lee HW, Lee JS, Ahn SH. Hepatitis B virus cure: targets and future therapies. Int J Mol Sci 2020;22(1). https://doi.org/10.3390/ijms22010213.
28. Centers for Disease Control and Prevention. Hepatitis D. Updated June 22, 2020. https://www.cdc.gov/hepatitis/hdv/index.htm. [Accessed 16 April 2022].
29. Yurdaydin C, Idilman R, Bozkaya H, et al. Natural history and treatment of chronic delta hepatitis. J Viral Hepat 2010;17(11):749–56.
30. Rizzetto M, Verme G, Recchia S, et al. Chronic hepatitis in carriers of hepatitis B surface antigen, with intrahepatic expression of the delta antigen. an active and progressive disease unresponsive to immunosuppressive treatment. Ann Intern Med 1983;98(4):437–41.
31. Wedemeyer H, Negro F. Devil hepatitis D: an orphan disease or largely underdiagnosed? Gut 2019;68(3):381–2.
32. Miao Z, Zhang S, Ou X, et al. Estimating the global prevalence, disease progression, and clinical outcome of hepatitis delta virus infection. J Iinfect Dis 2020;221(10):1677–87.
33. Stockdale AJ, Kreuels B, Henrion MYR, et al. The global prevalence of hepatitis D virus infection: systematic review and meta-analysis. J Hepatol 2020;73(3):523–32.

34. Chen HY, Shen DT, Ji DZ, et al. Prevalence and burden of hepatitis D virus infection in the global population: a systematic review and meta-analysis. Gut 2019; 68(3):512–21.

35. Da BL, Heller T, Koh C. Hepatitis D infection: from initial discovery to current investigational therapies. Gastroenterol Rep (Oxf) 2019;7(4):231–45.

36. Kushner T, Serper M, Kaplan DE. Delta hepatitis within the Veterans Affairs Medical System in the United States: prevalence, risk factors, and outcomes. J Hepatol 2015;63(3):586–92.

37. Gish RG, Yi DH, Kane S, et al. Coinfection with hepatitis B and D: epidemiology, prevalence and disease in patients in Northern California. J Gastroenterol Hepatol 2013;28(9):1521–5.

38. Kucirka LM, Farzadegan H, Feld JJ, et al. Prevalence, correlates, and viral dynamics of hepatitis delta among injection drug users. J Infect Dis 2010;202(6): 845–52.

39. Ahn J, Gish RG. Hepatitis D virus: a call to screening. Gastroenterol Hepatol (N Y) 2014;10(10):647–86.

40. Patel EU, Thio CL, Boon D, et al. Prevalence of hepatitis B and hepatitis D virus infections in the United States, 2011-2016. Clin Infect Dis 2019;69(4):709–12.

41. Wedemeyer H, Yurdaydin C, Dalekos GN, et al. Peginterferon plus adefovir versus either drug alone for hepatitis delta. N Engl J Med 2011;364(4):322–31.

42. Heidrich B, Manns MP, Wedemeyer H. Treatment options for hepatitis delta virus infection. Curr Infect Dis Rep 2013;15(1):31–8.

Coronavirus Disease-2019 and Implications on the Liver

Patrick T. Campbell, MD, Oren K. Fix, MD, MSc*

KEYWORDS

• Cirrhosis • Immunosuppression • SARS-CoV-2 • Transplant • Vaccination

KEY POINTS

- The coronavirus disease-2019 (COVID-19) pandemic has had a substantial impact on patients with chronic liver disease (CLD) and liver transplantation (LT) recipients.
- The management of many CLD has been significantly altered by the COVID-19 pandemic.
- Vaccination against COVID-19 protects patients with CLD and LT recipients from adverse outcomes and is safe in these patients.
- Vaccine efficacy may be reduced in LT recipients and other immunosuppressed patients.

INTRODUCTION

Severe acute respiratory syndrome coronavirus 2 (SARS-CoV-2) is a novel coronavirus that is responsible for causing coronavirus disease-2019 (COVID-19). SARS-CoV-2 was first detected in humans in late 2019 and spread to become a worldwide pandemic. This virus is most similar to the beta-coronaviruses, SARS-CoV and Middle East respiratory syndrome coronavirus (MERS-CoV), that were responsible for the SARS outbreak in 2002 to 2003 and the MERS outbreak in 2012, respectively. SARS-CoV-2 primarily causes upper respiratory tract infections and pneumonia. Severe cases can lead to acute respiratory distress syndrome and death. Although the lung manifestations are the most common and most severe, SARS-CoV-2 has effects on other organs including the liver and gastrointestinal tract. The aim of this article is to review the effects of SARS-CoV-2 on the liver and how COVID-19 and the resulting pandemic have altered the outcomes and management of chronic liver diseases (CLDs) and liver transplantation (LT).

Division of Gastroenterology and Hepatology, University of North Carolina School of Medicine, Burnett-Womack Building, Campus Box 7584, Chapel Hill, NC 27599-7584, USA
* Corresponding author.
E-mail address: oren.fix@unc.edu

Clin Liver Dis 27 (2023) 27–45
https://doi.org/10.1016/j.cld.2022.08.003
1089-3261/23/© 2022 Elsevier Inc. All rights reserved.

EFFECTS OF CORONAVIRUS DISEASE-2019 ON THE LIVER
Coronavirus Disease-2019 and Abnormal Liver Biochemistries

Abnormalities in liver biochemistries are common in patients with COVID-19, with a highly variable prevalence of 14% to 83% in hospitalized patients and occurring more frequently in severe COVID-19.[1–5] Liver biochemical abnormalities are most commonly characterized as mild elevations of alanine transaminase (ALT) and aspartate transaminase (AST) (<5 times the upper limit of normal [xULN]). Bilirubin is usually normal or only slightly elevated and alkaline phosphatase/gamma-glutamyl transferase elevations are uncommon (occurring in 6% and 21% of patients, respectively).[6] AST levels do not correlate with markers of muscle breakdown (creatinine kinase) or systemic inflammation (C-reactive protein and ferritin), suggesting that elevations seen in the setting of COVID-19 may be due to direct liver injury.[7] However, the incidence of liver biochemical abnormalities in patients with COVID-19 does not seem to be associated with the presence of preexisting CLD.[8] The aminotransferase elevation in COVID-19 is often AST-predominant, which is similar to alcohol-related liver disease and ischemic hepatitis.[7] The pattern of AST-predominant aminotransferase elevation has also been associated with COVID-19 disease severity.[4] The reason for AST predominance is unclear but could be related to hepatic hypoperfusion from COVID-19-induced microthrombotic disease[9] or systemic hypoxia. The fact that similar AST-predominant elevations were reported during the 2009 influenza H1N1 outbreak could support the hypothesis that systemic hypoxia is the underlying driver of this liver enzyme pattern.[10] Low albumin levels in the setting of COVID-19 can also be seen and correlate with more severe COVID-19.[11] Severe liver injury, defined as elevations in total bilirubin and/or evidence of synthetic dysfunction, is uncommon but associated with poorer clinical outcomes.[5] Given the frequency of elevated liver biochemistries in patients hospitalized with COVID-19, it is recommended that liver biochemistries be monitored regularly in this patient population.[12]

There can be many reasons for elevated liver biochemistries in patients with COVID-19, including muscle breakdown in the setting of myositis or cardiac injury, direct hepatic infection with SARS-CoV-2, hepatic ischemia caused by hypotension or thrombosis, cytokine release syndrome/immune-mediated injury, post-COVID cholangiopathy, and drug-induced liver injury (DILI) (**Fig. 1**). Given the broad differential, determining the exact cause of the elevated liver biochemistries in a patient with COVID-19 can be challenging and the cause is often multifactorial. **Fig. 2** offers a proposed algorithm for the evaluation of abnormal liver tests in the patient with COVID-19.

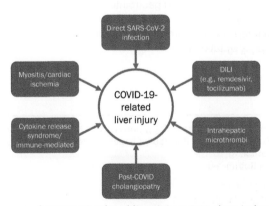

Fig. 1. Potential causes of COVID-19-related liver injury. DILI, drug-induced liver injury.

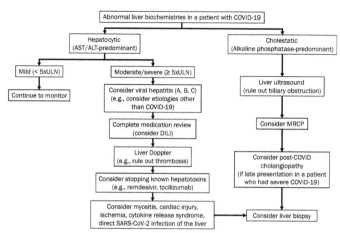

Fig. 2. Algorithm for the evaluation of abnormal liver biochemistries in the patient with COVID-19. DILI, drug-induced liver injury; MRCP, magnetic resonance cholangiopancreatography; ULN, upper limit of normal.

Direct Hepatic Infection via Angiotensin-Converting Enzyme 2 and/or Dipeptidyl Peptidase 4

SARS-CoV-2 binds to cells using angiotensin-converting enzyme 2 (ACE2) as a receptor and is subsequently internalized.[13] In the liver, ACE2 is found on cholangiocytes, sinusoidal epithelial cells, and hepatocytes. Direct viral infection of hepatocytes and cholangiocytes is one potential mechanism for COVID-19-induced hepatic injury because of the presence of ACE2 on these cells. Gene expression of ACE2 is greatest in cholangiocytes with levels that are comparable to alveolar type 2 cells in the lung.[14] Autopsy results from patients with COVID-19 have shown the presence of SARS-CoV-2 within hepatocytes confirming that hepatic infection by SARS-CoV-2 does occur,[15] likely via ACE2. Hepatic ACE2 levels are significantly upregulated in several CLDs including hepatitis C virus (HCV) (30-fold increase)[16] and nonalcoholic steatohepatitis (NASH) (compared with those with simple steatosis),[17] potentially predisposing these patients to more frequent and/or significant liver injury caused by COVID-19.

Another enzyme that may be responsible for direct hepatic insult from COVID-19 is dipeptidyl peptidase-4 (DPP-4). MERS-CoV is known to use DPP-4 as a receptor for cell entry and SARS-CoV-2 can also use DPP-4 as a receptor.[18] DPP-4 is found in most organs but is present in particularly high levels in the liver. It is often upregulated in diabetes and the metabolic syndrome,[19] which are frequently present in NASH. DPP-4 may also play a role in hepatic fibrosis.[20] Although these findings may suggest a possible mechanism of direct COVID-19-related liver injury, whether DPP-4 is truly responsible for elevated liver biochemistries in patients with COVID-19 is still unproven.

Thrombosis and Ischemia

Another possible mechanism of liver injury during COVID-19 is due to a pro-thrombotic state leading to microthrombi and resulting ischemia. It has been well documented that COVID-19 produces a hypercoagulable state that increases the risk of thrombosis and microvascular thrombosis.[21] Autopsy studies of patients who died from COVID-19 have discovered the presence of microthrombi in several organs including the liver. In one study, liver biopsy samples from 48 patients who died from severe COVID-19 revealed portal venous and sinusoidal microthombi in all patients.[9] A meta-analysis of several autopsy studies found a lower, but still significant, prevalence of hepatic vascular thrombosis (29%).[22] This study also reported cases of hepatic venous outflow obstruction and phlebosclerosis of the portal vein.

Immune-Mediated Injury

COVID-19 is known to cause a significant pro-inflammatory response and cytokine release syndrome; therefore, an immune-mediated injury may be contributing to elevated liver biochemistries in patients with COVID-19. Patients with COVID-19 with elevated liver biochemistries are more likely to have fever, higher levels of pro-inflammatory markers (C-reactive protein and procalcitonin), and higher lactate dehydrogenase.[23] However, further study is needed to determine if COVID-19 truly causes an immune-mediated liver injury.

Post-Coronavirus Disease Cholangiopathy

Cholangiopathy has been described as a rare, late liver-related complication of severe COVID-19.[24–26] In one study of 2047 patients who were hospitalized with COVID-19, 12 patients with severe COVID-19 developed cholangiopathy.[25] The imaging and histologic findings in these patients were similar to the previously described secondary sclerosing cholangitis in critically ill patients (SSC-CIP).[27] Typical magnetic resonance cholangiopancreatography findings in these patients included beading of intrahepatic bile ducts and bile duct wall thickening with enhancement. Several patients underwent liver biopsy that showed large bile duct obstruction without bile duct loss. The average time to cholangiopathy diagnosis was 118 days after initial COVID-19 diagnosis. Five of these patients were eventually evaluated for LT because of persistent jaundice, hepatic dysfunction, and/or recurrent episodes of bacterial cholangitis, and one did eventually undergo LT.[25] The underlying pathogenesis explaining why post-COVID cholangiopathy occurs is not currently understood and further study in this area is needed.

Effect of Coronavirus Disease-2019-Directed Therapies on the Liver

DILI is a frequent cause of elevated liver biochemistries in hospitalized patients with COVID-19, including two COVID-19-directed therapies, remdesivir, and tocilizumab, that have been implicated as possible causes of DILI in patients with COVID-19.

Remdesivir, a viral RNA polymerase inhibitor, was one of the first drugs to show efficacy against COVID-19. The earliest studies of compassionate-use remdesivir showed that elevated liver biochemistries were the most frequently reported adverse event. Compared with placebo, patients receiving remdesivir more frequently had treatment discontinued for elevated transaminases or bilirubin. However, these studies were not adequately powered to determine if a significant difference existed.[28] Subsequently, a large randomized controlled trial of remdesivir use in COVID-19 showed no difference in liver biochemistries between treatment and control groups.[29] Nonetheless, it is still recommended to avoid remdesivir in patients with ALT greater than 5 xULN and it should be discontinued if ALT increases above this level while on treatment.

Tocilizumab, an IL-6 antagonist that inhibits the pro-inflammatory cytokine cascade, has been used to treat COVID-19. Tocilizumab-induced liver injury has previously been documented in patients receiving it for rheumatoid arthritis, although these events are very rare.[30] There have also been several case reports of apparent tocilizumab-DILI in patients with COVID-19, with one patient having aminotransferase elevations greater than 40 xULN[31]; however, these cases are also very rare.

Tocilizumab is not recommended in patients with aminotransferase elevations greater than 5 xULN.

ALCOHOL-RELATED LIVER DISEASE AND THE CORONAVIRUS DISEASE-2019 PANDEMIC

In the years before the start of the COVID-19 pandemic, alcohol consumption and mortality from alcohol-associated liver disease were already on the rise.[32] During the COVID-19 pandemic this rise has continued and even accelerated. Stay-at-home orders early in the pandemic led to social isolation, loss of support systems including addiction treatment programs, disruptions in work and education, and easier access to alcohol (eg, online, takeout), all factors that likely contributed to a significant increase in alcohol consumption and alcohol-associated liver disease during the pandemic.[33] This manifested in drastic increases in listings for LT (7% increase) and LT (10% increase) for alcohol-associated liver disease.[34] Transplant listing and LT for severe alcohol-associated hepatitis alone have also rapidly increased by over 50%, likely because of an increased burden of alcohol-related liver disease during the pandemic but also due to an unrelated nationwide shift away from strict policies requiring at least 6 months of alcohol abstinence before consideration of LT.

CORONAVIRUS DISEASE-2019 OUTCOMES IN LIVER DISEASE
Chronic Liver Disease and Cirrhosis

Several studies have shown that patients with CLD are not more likely to be diagnosed with COVID-19 [2,35] and one study indicated that patients with cirrhosis might actually have a lower risk of testing positive for SARS-CoV-2.[36] This is likely due to increased patient adherence to public health measures such as social distancing because it is unlikely that cirrhosis provides a protective effect. However, once patients with pre-existing liver disease of any etiology are diagnosed with COVID-19, they have higher rates of mortality than those without liver disease. Respiratory failure is the leading cause of death in patients with CLD and COVID-19, followed by liver-related causes.[8,37]

The same has been shown in patients with cirrhosis even after adjusting for covariates (eg, etiology of liver disease, race, comorbidities, geographic region).[38] Outcomes seem to be correlated with severity of pre-existing cirrhosis, with odds ratio (OR) of death for Child-Pugh (CP)-A 1.90, CP-B 4.14 and CP-C 9.32.[37] Outcomes for patients with decompensated cirrhosis and COVID-19 are extremely poor, with mortality rates as high as 80% for patients who require intensive care unit (ICU) admission.[37] Although early mortality rates in patients with cirrhosis and COVID-19 are high, the rates of death and readmission at 90 days for patients who survive the acute insult return to baseline risk.[39] Therefore, COVID-19 does not seem to result in long-term progression of liver disease outside of the acute infection period.

Viral Hepatitis

In 2017, the World Health Organization released the first Global Hepatitis Report and set a goal of eliminating viral hepatitis by 2030.[40] Unfortunately, the necessary diversion of limited health care resources toward COVID-19 efforts limited the identification of new hepatitis B virus (HBV) and HCV infections and also limited access to treatment. This delay in viral hepatitis elimination and treatment because of the COVID-19 pandemic will certainly result in worse long-term viral hepatitis outcomes, with many patients progressing to cirrhosis and developing its accompanying complications such as hepatocellular carcinoma (HCC). A modeling study of 100 countries predicted that a 1-year delay in the diagnosis of HCV could lead to an additional 44,800 cases of HCC and 72,300 deaths from HCV worldwide by 2030.[41] Fortunately, the presence of HBV or HCV alone is not associated with COVID-19 mortality.[42] In addition, antiviral therapy for HBV or HCV has not been associated with worsened COVID-19 outcomes.

Nonalcoholic Steatohepatitis

It has been well documented that older age, obesity and diabetes are associated with worsened COVID-19 outcomes.[35] Given obesity and diabetes are often comorbid with NASH, there has been concern that patients with NASH are at increased risk of poor COVID-19-related outcomes. However, whether NASH independent of comorbidities increases the risk of severe COVID-19 and death is unclear. Several studies have suggested this might be true: nonalcoholic fatty liver disease (NAFLD) has been associated with worsened COVID-19 outcomes independent of obesity and other comorbidities.[43,44] However, a large international cohort of 745 patients with cirrhosis and/or CLD failed to show an increased risk of mortality for NAFLD patients with COVID-19 (HR 1.01, 95% CI 0.57–1.79).[37]

Autoimmune Hepatitis

There has also been concern that patients with autoimmune hepatitis (AIH) would be at increased risk of COVID-19-related morbidity and mortality. Interestingly, despite the use of immunosuppression, patients with AIH seem to have similar outcomes compared with patients with other CLD.[45] Furthermore, AIH patients seem to have equivalent rates of COVID-19-related mortality when compared with the general population, and immunosuppression was not shown to be an independent risk factor for mortality or severe COVID-19.[45,46]

Liver Transplant Recipients

Given their immunosuppressed state, it was feared that LT recipients would be at increased risk for severe COVID-19 and death. LT recipients are diagnosed with COVID-19 more frequently than non-transplant recipients.[47,48] However, this is likely because of closer monitoring and a lower threshold for testing in this patient population as opposed to an increased risk of SARS-CoV-2 infection per se. LT recipients do seem to report more frequent gastrointestinal symptoms, with diarrhea occurring in 30% to 40%,[49,50] but rates of elevated liver biochemistries are similar between LT and non-LT recipients.[49,51] LT recipients are also more likely to have chronic kidney disease, type 2 diabetes mellitus, and obesity, which are well known risk factors for worse COVID-19-related outcomes. Yet, the studies to date have been conflicting. Several studies have reported high mortality rates in solid organ transplant recipients with COVID-19.[50,52] However, after controlling for covariates including comorbidities, several other studies have suggested that LT recipients may not be at an increased risk of severe COVID-19 or death compared with non-LT recipients.[47,49] This would be consistent with studies from the prior novel coronavirus outbreaks (SARS and MERS) that showed LT recipients were not at increased risk of morbidity and mortality compared with the general population.[53] The suggestion of similar clinical outcomes between LT recipients and non-transplant recipients could be explained by the theorized protective effects of immunosuppression against a SARS-CoV-2-induced severe inflammatory host response, which is thought to be a primary driver in severe COVID-19.[54] This is supported by data showing that high dose dexamethasone improves mortality in patients with severe COVID-19.[55]

MANAGEMENT OF CHRONIC LIVER DISEASE DURING THE CORONAVIRUS DISEASE-2019 PANDEMIC

The optimal management of CLD during the COVID-19 pandemic is continually evolving as new data become available. In addition, management varies based on the presence or absence of active SAR-CoV-2 infection and on the underlying liver disease etiology (**Table 1**).

Autoimmune Hepatitis

Without coronavirus disease-2019

Given the risk of a flare/relapse with reduction or discontinuation of immunosuppression,[56] providers should not adjust baseline immunosuppression for AIH in hopes of preventing COVID-19-related morbidity and mortality. A new diagnosis of AIH or a flare of existing AIH should be treated as clinically appropriate despite the risk of SARS-CoV-2 infection.

Table 1
Management of CLD during the COVID-19 pandemic

Etiology	Without COVID-19	With COVID-19
Autoimmune hepatitis	• Do not preemptively reduce immunosuppression • Treat new diagnosis or flare as clinically appropriate	Mild COVID-19: • Do not reduce immunosuppression Moderate/severe COVID-19: • Consider reducing immunosuppression by 25%-50% • Consider reducing or stopping antimetabolite (eg, azathioprine, mycophenolate)
Chronic viral hepatitis	No change(ie, start or continue antiviral therapy as clinically appropriate)	HBV: • Initiate or continue treatment if indicated based on current HBV treatment guidelines • Consider HBV prophylaxis if treating COVID-19 with immunosuppression (eg, dexamethasone, tocilizumab) HCV: • Continue HCV therapy if already started • Postpone initiation of HCV therapy until after recovery from COVID-19
NASH	No change	No change
PBC	No change	No change
PSC	No change	No change
ALD	No change	No change

Abbreviations: ALD, alcohol-associated liver disease; CLD, chronic liver disease; HBV, hepatitis B virus; HCV, hepatitis C virus; NASH, nonalcoholic steatohepatitis; PBC, primary biliary cholangitis; PSC, primary sclerosing cholangitis.

With coronavirus disease-2019

Given similar COVID-19-related outcomes in patients with AIH on immunosuppression compared with the general population,[45] providers should not routinely reduce immunosuppression in the setting of a new COVID-19 diagnosis. The severity of COVID-19 should first be considered to determine the best next steps. For outpatients with asymptomatic or mild COVID-19, immunosuppression should not be adjusted. For patients with moderate to severe COVID-19 (ie, hospitalized and/or ICU admission), the patient's AIH disease history (such as frequency of prior relapses) and fibrosis stage should be considered. For instance, a flare of AIH in a patient with cirrhosis/advanced fibrosis could result in hepatic decompensation; therefore, the threshold for reducing immunosuppression in these patients should be higher. If the decision is made to reduce immunosuppression, baseline doses may be reduced by 25% to 50%. The patient should subsequently be monitored closely for a AIH flare by checking liver enzymes daily in the hospitalized patient and every 1 to 2 weeks once the patient is discharged. For patients on antimetabolites such as azathioprine or mycophenolate with neutropenia and/or lymphopenia associated with COVID-19, the antimetabolite dose should be reduced or stopped and a white blood cell count with differential should be monitored every 1 to 2 weeks.

Chronic Viral Hepatitis

Without coronavirus disease-2019

Antiviral therapies have not been shown to increase the risk of severe COVID-19. Therefore, antiviral therapy can be safely started and continued in HBV and HCV patients without COVID-19.

With coronavirus disease-2019

Given antiviral therapy does not worsen COVID-19 outcomes, continuation of antiviral therapy for patients with HBV and HCV is also recommended for those with SARS-CoV-2 infection. As initiation of therapy for HCV is not urgent, initiation of HCV therapy for patients with COVID-19 should be postponed until the patient has recovered from COVID-19.[12] HBV therapy should be initiated despite active SARS-CoV-2 infection if indicated based on current HBV treatment guidelines. Given the risk of reactivation of HBV with immunosuppression, patients started on immunosuppression for COVID-19 with medications such as glucocorticoids or tocilizumab should be considered for HBV prophylaxis.[12,57,58]

Other Chronic Liver Diseases (Nonalcoholic Steatohepatitis, Alcohol-Associated Liver Disease, Primary Biliary Cholangitis, and Primary Sclerosing Cholangitis)

The management strategies for many CLDs including NASH, alcohol-associated liver disease, primary biliary cholangitis (PBC) and primary sclerosing cholangitis (PSC) have not been significantly altered by the COVID-19 pandemic. Patients with NASH should continue to be advised on risk factor control (diabetes, hyperlipidemia, and hypertension) and lifestyle changes to promote weight loss, although it should be acknowledged that the pandemic has made exercise and healthy eating habits more challenging for many. Patients with severe alcohol-associated hepatitis can be considered for corticosteroid treatment if indicated. Routine screening for colorectal cancer, gallbladder carcinoma and cholangiocarcinoma for patients with PSC should continue. Patients with PBC on treatment (such as ursodiol) should continue on this even if they develop SARS-CoV-2 infection.

Telemedicine/Delivery of Care

Telemedicine, which is the delivery of health care from afar using technology, previously had slow uptake because of restrictive regulations, lack of reimbursement, lack of widespread Internet infrastructure, and resistance to change.[59] However, shortly after the pandemic began there was a drastic increase in telemedicine use to help with mitigation efforts to slow the spread of COVID-19.[60] Many restrictions on telemedicine services were lifted along with changes in reimbursement. As the pandemic progresses, it remains unseen how the delivery and use of telemedicine will continue to evolve. For liver-related care, telemedicine offers particular promise in the delivery of subspecialty hepatology care to patients in rural areas, those with limited transportation and financial means, and incarcerated persons. For example, the effort to eliminate viral hepatitis will likely need to rely heavily on telemedicine to reach these populations.[61] However, there are many patients with CLD with socioeconomic disparities that may limit their access to high-speed Internet resulting in inadequate access to telemedicine.[62] There will need to be a specific focus on improving Internet infrastructure, expanding access to computers and mobile devices, and education to improve technological competence, to ensure that these populations have equitable access to telemedicine.

CORONAVIRUS DISEASE-2019 VACCINATION

Patients with CLD have an increased risk of COVID-19 morbidity and mortality and should be prioritized for COVID-19 vaccination and booster doses.[63] All of the available SARS-CoV-2 vaccines, including the messenger ribonucleic acid (mRNA) (Pfizer-BioNTech, Moderna) and adenoviral vector vaccines (Johnson & Johnson [J&J], AstraZeneca, Sputnik), are safe for patients with CLD and there are no contraindications for their use in this patient population.[64–66] Thus, patients should be vaccinated as soon as they are eligible and a vaccine is available to them.[64] COVID-19 vaccination does not require delaying or discontinuing therapy for any CLD such as antiviral therapy for HBV/HCV or immunosuppression for AIH. Routine non-COVID-19 vaccines (such as vaccination against hepatitis A or HBV) also do not need to be delayed while patients are receiving the COVID-19 vaccine series and can be given as scheduled. For further guidance regarding COVID-19 vaccination in patients with liver disease, AASLD has created an expert panel consensus statement that will be continually updated as new data arise.[63]

Cirrhosis/Chronic Liver Disease

Patients with cirrhosis have been shown to have impaired responses to non-COVID-19 vaccines such as pneumococcus and HBV, likely due to immune dysfunction seen in cirrhosis.[67,68] Although there are limited data currently on the efficacy of COVD-19 vaccines in patients with CLD, the available data suggest a similar impaired but still significantly protective response to COVID-19 vaccines. A large study from the Veterans Affairs system propensity matched 20,037 patients with CLD who had received one dose of an mRNA vaccine (Moderna or Pfizer-BioNTech) with 20,037 control patients who had not been vaccinated. At 28 days after one dose, there was a 64% reduction in SARS-CoV-2 infections and 100% reduction in hospitalization and death in patients with CLD. A second dose provided additional protection with a 78% reduction in SARS-CoV-2 infections and 100% protection against hospitalization and death. This contrasts with a 94%-95% reduction in SARS-CoV-2 infections after two doses of an mRNA vaccine in the general population.[65,66] The severity of liver disease is also associated with impaired response to vaccination. Vaccinated patients with decompensated cirrhosis had only a 50% reduction in new SARS-CoV-2 infections compared with 66% in patients with compensated cirrhosis.[69]

Liver Transplantation Recipients

Data on COVID-19 immunization in LT recipients have shown the vaccines to be safe and effective at preventing hospitalization and death.[63] Available data do not show an increased risk of alloimmunity and graft rejection.[70] It is important to note that none of the available vaccines contain live SARS-CoV-2; therefore, replication of SARS-CoV-2 after vaccination is not possible even in immunocompromised patients. However, compared with immunocompetent individuals, LT recipients have lower levels of anti-spike antibody production after COVID-19 vaccination and a quicker decline in antibody levels over time.[71] This is similar to prior studies that have shown LT recipients have a poor response to non-COVID-19 vaccinations.[70] Risk factors for poor antibody formation after COVID-19 vaccination in this population include older age, chronic kidney disease, use of high dose steroids and use of mycophenolate mofetil.[72] Despite this, it is not recommended to reduce immunosuppression to improve immune response to COVID-19 vaccination given the risk of acute cellular rejection.[63] The antibody response from mRNA COVID-19 vaccination can be improved with additional doses.[73,74] As a result, current guidelines recommend a primary series of three doses for the mRNA vaccines in immunocompromised patients including LT recipients followed by one or more booster doses (**Table 2**).[63] For patients who received the J&J vaccine, the primary series should consist of a second dose of the J&J vaccine or a dose of an mRNA vaccine followed by one or more booster doses. Given that antibody formation after vaccination is greater for patients with cirrhosis compared with post LT patients, candidates for LT should be vaccinated before transplant whenever possible.[63,75] Potential live liver donors should also be encouraged to undergo

---

Table 2
General guidelines for COVID-19 vaccination for adults in the United States with CLD and LT recipients

	Number/Manufacturer ofPrimary Series	Booster
CLD	2 Pfizer-BioNTech mRNA*or*2 Moderna mRNA*or*2 Novavax adjuvanted*or*1 J&J/Janssen adenoviral vector[a]	Bivalent Pfizer-BioNTech or Moderna mRNA ≥2 months after primary series
AIH on immunosuppression	3 Pfizer-BioNTech mRNA*or*3 Moderna mRNA*or*2 Novavax adjuvanted*or*1 J&J/Janssen adenoviral vector followed by any mRNA vaccine[a]	Bivalent Pfizer-BioNTech or Moderna mRNA ≥2 months after primary series
LT recipients	3 Pfizer-BioNTech mRNA*or*3 Moderna mRNA*or*2 Novavax adjuvanted*or*1 J&J/Janssen adenoviral vector followed by any mRNA vaccine[a]	Bivalent Pfizer-BioNTech or Moderna mRNA ≥2 months after primary series

Abbreviations: AIH, autoimmune hepatitis; CLD, chronic liver disease; LT, liver transplant
See CDC website for additional details, including dose intervals and pediatric recommendations: https://www.cdc.gov/vaccines/covid-19/clinical-considerations/interim-considerations-us.html.
[a] Janssen COVID-19 vaccine should only be used in certain limited situations; mRNA primary vaccine series preferred whenever possible

vaccination before donation. Even if LT is likely to happen before completion of the vaccine series, COVID-19 vaccination should continue after transplantation. Any additional vaccine doses that need to be completed post-LT can be given at the earliest appropriate interval following transplant (around 4 weeks' post-LT). If COVID-19 vaccination cannot be started before transplant, the optimal timing for vaccination is likely at least 3 months post-LT when immunosuppression is lower to allow for better antibody formation; however, it is possible to begin vaccination as early as 4 weeks post-LT.[63]

Table 2 shows general guidelines for COVID-19 vaccination in adults with CLD and LT recipients. Recommendations for vaccination in LT recipients are likely to change as new data become available. Additional booster doses may be recommended for both transplant recipients and the general population as immunity naturally wanes and new viral variants emerge. Check the CDC website for the latest available recommendations: https://www.cdc.gov/vaccines/covid-19/clinical-considerations/interim-considerations-us.html#immunocompromised.

Liver Transplantation Candidates

COVID-19 vaccines have been proven to be safe and effective at preventing hospitalization and death in patients with cirrhosis and in LT recipients.[63] When possible, vaccination should occur before transplant due to better antibody formation and protection against poor outcomes after vaccination in patients with cirrhosis compared with LT recipients.[75] Many transplant centers have required COVID-19 and other vaccinations before listing for liver transplant. These policies are clinically and ethically justified but remain at the discretion of each transplant center.[76]

Autoimmune Hepatitis

Patients with AIH on immunosuppression have also been shown to have a poor response to vaccinations against non-COVID-19 diseases.[70] Early data on COVID-19 vaccination for patients on immunosuppression also indicate an impaired immune response in this population.[77] Therefore, it is currently recommended that immunosuppressed patients, including patients with AIH on immunosuppression, receive a three-dose primary series of an mRNA vaccine plus one or more booster doses (see **Table 2**).[78]

There have been several case reports of a rare AIH-like liver injury following COVID-19 vaccination.[79–81] A systematic review by Chow and colleagues summarized the existing case reports and series that included 32 patients with an AIH-like syndrome following an mRNA or Oxford-AstraZeneca COVID-19 vaccine.[82] Several of these patients did not meet criteria for AIH and likely just had hepatocellular or cholestatic DILI to the vaccine without autoimmune features. There was also a small subset of patients (n = 4) who had a prior diagnosis of AIH that was in remission before receiving the vaccine and then developed a flare following COVID-19 vaccination.[83] Given the low incidence, it has not been determined whether these rare events are simply coincidental or causally related to the vaccine. This rare potential risk should not discourage COVID-19 vaccination, even in those with preexisting AIH or CLD.

LIVER TRANSPLANTATION AND CORONAVIRUS DISEASE-2019
Severe Acute Respiratory Syndrome Coronavirus 2-Positive Liver Transplantation Recipient

LT recipients require high doses of immunosuppression immediately post-transplant to prevent rejection and there is significant concern for worsened post-LT outcomes if a transplant recipient were to become infected with SARS-CoV-2 at the time of transplant. As a result it is recommended that all recipients be tested for SARS-CoV-2 before transplant.[12] There have been several reports of successful living donor LT in SARS-CoV-2-positive recipients after a minimum of 14 days from positive SARS-CoV-2 PCR.[12] However, available data suggest that the risk of postoperative morbidity and mortality related to recent COVID-19 can remain high for much longer than 14 days after acute infection and seems to remain particularly elevated for up to 7 weeks post-infection.[12,84] Therefore, except in extreme circumstances, patients with active/recent COVID-19 should not undergo LT.[12] The specific circumstances and urgency of the recipient should be considered when deciding whether to proceed with LT.

Severe Acute Respiratory Syndrome Coronavirus 2-Positive Donor

If an organ from a SARS-CoV-2-positive donor is transplanted into a SARS-CoV-2-negative recipient, there is a theoretic risk of SARS-CoV-2 transmission from the donor to recipient. To date, all of the reported cases of SARS-CoV-2 transmission from a COVID-19-positive donor have occurred in lung transplantation[85] and there have been no proven or suspected cases of donor-to-recipient SARS-CoV-2 transmission in non-lung transplants.[86] In fact, several case reports have described the successful use of SARS-CoV-2 positive donors without documented transmission to the transplant recipient in non-lung solid organ transplant.[87–91] Given the limited data that exist, no recommendation regarding the risk of SARS-CoV-2 transmission to the recipient can be made.[12]

Given the concerns about possible donor-to-recipient transmission, it is recommended that all potential donors be tested for SARS-CoV-2 before LT.[12] However, SARS-CoV-2 PCR may remain positive for months after resolution of infection despite a patient no longer being infectious. Although a lack of infiltrates on chest imaging or a SARS-CoV-2 diagnosis greater than 10 days earlier may indicate inactive infection, it can often be hard to differentiate between active and inactive infection.[12] The cycle time (number of amplification cycles needed to produce a positive PCR test) may be helpful to differentiate active from inactive infection.[92] Low cycle times reflect higher viral load, whereas high cycle times reflect lower viral load, possibly indicating inactive infection.

The decision to proceed with transplantation using a SARS-CoV-2-positive donor should consider the severity and timing of COVID-19 in the potential donor and the urgency of the potential recipient. Donor organ quality should also be considered independently from the risk of donor-to-recipient viral transmission.

Management of the Liver Transplantation Recipient without Coronavirus Disease-2019

Given the risk of acute cellular rejection, maintenance immunosuppression should be continued and the doses should not be lowered. Patients who develop acute rejection should also continue to receive the standard of care with high dose immunosuppression to preserve graft function.[93]

Management of the Liver Transplantation Recipient with Coronavirus Disease-2019

For LT recipients with an active SARS-CoV-2 infection, the decision to modify immunosuppression and dosing should be individualized based on history of rejection, the risk of future rejection, length of time post-LT and the severity of COVID-19. Tacrolimus has been associated with better survival in transplant recipients with COVID-19 and generally should not be decreased or stopped.[94] Mycophenolate, however, has been found to be an independent risk factor for severe COVID-19 in LT recipients and decreasing or stopping it is a reasonable approach to managing LT recipients with moderate/severe COVID-19.[47]

Outpatient/Mild Coronavirus Disease-2019 Management

Immunosuppression should not be adjusted for LT recipients with mild COVID-19. There are several treatment options available for patients who are diagnosed with COVID-19 including nirmatrelvir-ritonavir (Paxlovid), molnupiravir, monoclonal antibodies and remdesivir. Nirmatrelvir-ritonavir is a combination of oral protease inhibitors that blocks SARS-CoV-2 protease activity. In a randomized controlled trial, it was shown to be highly effective at reducing rates of hospitalization or death (89% reduction compared with placebo).[95] Nirmatrelvir-ritonavir is not recommended in patients with severe renal (eGFR 30 mL/min) or severe liver (CP-C) impairment. There are significant drug interactions with nirmatrelvir-ritonavir, especially calcineurin inhibitors, which may lead to dangerously high levels of these drugs in some transplant recipients. For patients who are not candidates for nirmatrelvir-ritonavir, other therapies that can be considered are monoclonal antibodies, remdesivir and molnupiravir.

Inpatient/Moderate–Severe Coronavirus Disease-2019 Management

Given the association of antimetabolite medications and worsened COVID-19 outcomes, it is recommended that doses of azathioprine or mycophenolate should be lowered in moderate to severe COVID-19, including patients hospitalized for COVID-19.[12] Glucocorticoids may be beneficial in severe COVID-19 and have not been shown to worsen outcomes; therefore, immunosuppression consisting of glucocorticoids should not be routinely adjusted.[96] In patients who develop neutropenia and/or lymphopenia (absolute lymphocyte count <1000 cells/microL for adults) due to COVID-19, the dose of azathioprine or mycophenolate should be reduced and labs (white blood cell count with differential and liver biochemistries) should be checked every 1 to 2 weeks to monitor for rejection and improvement in neutropenia and/or lymphopenia.

SUMMARY

The COVID-19 pandemic has had a substantial impact on patients with CLD and LT recipients and has significantly altered the care of these patients. Vaccination against COVID-19 is effective at protecting patients with CLD and LT recipients from adverse outcomes and is safe in these patients; however, vaccine efficacy may be reduced in LT recipients and other immunosuppressed patients. COVID-19 has challenged the transplant community and the decisions about the use of potential donors with recent or current SARS-CoV-2 infection and when it is safe to proceed with LT in potential recipients with SARS-CoV-2 infection.

CLINICS CARE POINTS

- Compared to the general population, patients with chronic liver disease and liver transplant recipients are at a significantly increased risk of poor outcomes due to COVID-19.
- For patients without active COVID-19 infection who are on immunosuppression for autoimmune hepatitis or after liver transplantation, the doses of immunosuppressive medications should not be routinely altered in an attempt to prevent COVID-19 complications.
- In addition, flares of autoimmune hepatitis or episodes of post liver transplant rejection should be treated as clinically appropriate.

- Although patients with chronic liver disease and liver transplant recipients may have an impaired response to COVID-19 vaccination, vaccination in these patients has still been proven to be safe and effective at preventing morbidity and mortality due to COVID-19.
- Antibody formation after vaccination has been shown to be greater in patients with chronic liver disease as compared to liver transplant recipients, therefore COVID-19 vaccination prior to transplant should be prioritized.

DISCLOSURE

The authors have no relevant commercial or financial conflicts of interest and no funding was received for this article.

REFERENCES

1. Hundt MA, Deng Y, Ciarleglio MM, et al. Abnormal liver tests in COVID-19: a retrospective Observational cohort study of 1,827 patients in a Major U.S. Hospital Network. Hepatology 2020;72(4):1169–76.
2. Richardson S, Hirsch JS, Narasimhan M, et al. Presenting Characteristics, comorbidities, and outcomes among 5700 patients hospitalized with COVID-19 in the New York city area. JAMA 2020;323(20):2052–9.
3. Zhang C, Shi L, Wang FS. Liver injury in COVID-19: management and challenges. Lancet Gastroenterol Hepatol 2020;5(5):428–30.
4. Huang C, Wang Y, Li X, et al. Clinical features of patients infected with 2019 novel coronavirus in Wuhan, China. Lancet 2020;395(10223):497–506.
5. Phipps MM, Barraza LH, LaSota ED, et al. Acute liver injury in COVID-19: prevalence and association with clinical outcomes in a large U.S. Cohort. Hepatology 2020;72(3):807–17.
6. Kulkarni AV, Kumar P, Tevethia HV, et al. Systematic review with meta-analysis: liver manifestations and outcomes in COVID-19. Aliment Pharmacol Ther 2020; 52(4):584–99.
7. Bloom PP, Meyerowitz EA, Reinus Z, et al. Liver biochemistries in hospitalized patients with COVID-19. Hepatology 2021;73(3):890–900.
8. Singh S, Khan A. Clinical Characteristics and outcomes of coronavirus disease 2019 among patients with Preexisting liver disease in the United States: a multicenter Research Network study. Gastroenterology 2020;159(2):768–71.e3.
9. Sonzogni A, Previtali G, Seghezzi M, et al. Liver histopathology in severe COVID 19 respiratory failure is suggestive of vascular alterations. Liver Int 2020;40(9): 2110–6.
10. Papic N, Pangercic A, Vargovic M, et al. Liver involvement during influenza infection: perspective on the 2009 influenza pandemic. Influenza Other Respir Viruses 2012;6(3). e2-5.
11. Zhou F, Yu T, Du R, et al. Clinical course and risk factors for mortality of adult inpatients with COVID-19 in Wuhan, China: a retrospective cohort study. Lancet 2020;395(10229):1054–62.
12. Fix O, Fontana R, Bezerra J, et al. Clinical best Practice Advice for hepatology and liver transplant providers during the COVID-19 pandemic: AASLD expert panel consensus statement. Available at: http://www.aasld.org/ClinicalInsights. Accessed April 19, 2022.
13. Lan J, Ge J, Yu J, et al. Structure of the SARS-CoV-2 spike receptor-binding domain bound to the ACE2 receptor. Nature 2020;581(7807):215–20.

14. Pirola CJ, Sookoian S. SARS-CoV-2 virus and liver expression of host receptors: Putative mechanisms of liver involvement in COVID-19. Liver Int 2020;40(8): 2038–40.

15. Lagana SM, Kudose S, Iuga AC, et al. Hepatic pathology in patients dying of COVID-19: a series of 40 cases including clinical, histologic, and virologic data. Mod Pathol 2020;33(11):2147–55.

16. Paizis G, Tikellis C, Cooper ME, et al. Chronic liver injury in rats and humans up-regulates the novel enzyme angiotensin converting enzyme 2. Gut 2005;54(12): 1790–6.

17. Fondevila MF, Mercado-Gómez M, Rodríguez A, et al. Obese patients with NASH have increased hepatic expression of SARS-CoV-2 critical entry points. J Hepatol 2021;74(2):469–71.

18. Vankadari N, Wilce JA. Emerging WuHan (COVID-19) coronavirus: glycan shield and structure prediction of spike glycoprotein and its interaction with human CD26. Emerg Microbes Infect 2020;9(1):601–4.

19. Bassendine MF, Bridge SH, McCaughan GW, et al. COVID-19 and comorbidities: a role for dipeptidyl peptidase 4 (DPP4) in disease severity? J Diabetes 2020; 12(9):649–58.

20. Kaji K, Yoshiji H, Ikenaka Y, et al. Dipeptidyl peptidase-4 inhibitor attenuates hepatic fibrosis via suppression of activated hepatic stellate cell in rats. J Gastroenterol Mar 2014;49(3):481–91.

21. Connors JM, Levy JH. Thromboinflammation and the hypercoagulability of COVID-19. J Thromb Haemost 2020;18(7):1559–61.

22. Díaz LA, Idalsoaga F, Cannistra M, et al. High prevalence of hepatic steatosis and vascular thrombosis in COVID-19: a systematic review and meta-analysis of autopsy data. World J Gastroenterol 2020;26(48):7693–706.

23. Fan Z, Chen L, Li J, et al. Clinical features of COVID-19-related liver functional abnormality. Clin Gastroenterol Hepatol 2020;18(7):1561–6.

24. Roth NC, Kim A, Vitkovski T, et al. Post-COVID-19 cholangiopathy: a novel Entity. Am J Gastroenterol 2021;116(5):1077–82.

25. Faruqui S, Okoli FC, Olsen SK, et al. Cholangiopathy after severe COVID-19: clinical features and Prognostic Implications. Am J Gastroenterol 2021;116(7): 1414–25.

26. Durazo FA, Nicholas AA, Mahaffey JJ, et al. Post-Covid-19 cholangiopathy-A new indication for liver transplantation: a case report. Transplant Proc 2021;53(4): 1132–7.

27. Laurent L, Lemaitre C, Minello A, et al. Cholangiopathy in critically ill patients surviving beyond the intensive care period: a multicentre survey in liver units. Aliment Pharmacol Ther 2017;46(11–12):1070–6.

28. Montastruc F, Thuriot S, Durrieu G. Hepatic Disorders with the Use of remdesivir for coronavirus 2019. Clin Gastroenterol Hepatol 2020;18(12):2835–6.

29. Beigel JH, Tomashek KM, Dodd LE, et al. Remdesivir for the treatment of covid-19 - Final report. N Engl J Med 2020;383(19):1813–26.

30. Mahamid M, Mader R, Safadi R. Hepatotoxicity of tocilizumab and anakinra in rheumatoid arthritis: management decisions. Clin Pharm 2011;3:39–43.

31. Muhović D, Bojović J, Bulatović A, et al. First case of drug-induced liver injury associated with the use of tocilizumab in a patient with COVID-19. Liver Int 2020;40(8):1901–5.

32. Deutsch-Link S, Jiang Y, Peery AF, et al. Alcohol-associated liver disease mortality increased from 2017 to 2020 and accelerated during the COVID-19 pandemic. Clin Gastroenterol Hepatol 2022. https://doi.org/10.1016/j.cgh.2022.03.017.

33. Moon AM, Curtis B, Mandrekar P, et al. Alcohol-associated liver disease before and after COVID-19-an Overview and Call for Ongoing Investigation. Hepatol Commun 2021;5(9):1616–21.
34. Cholankeril G, Goli K, Rana A, et al. Impact of COVID-19 pandemic on liver transplantation and alcohol-associated liver disease in the USA. Hepatology 2021; 74(6):3316–29.
35. Williamson EJ, Walker AJ, Bhaskaran K, et al. Factors associated with COVID-19-related death using OpenSAFELY. Nature 2020;584(7821):430–6.
36. Ioannou GN, Liang PS, Locke E, et al. Cirrhosis and severe acute respiratory syndrome coronavirus 2 infection in US Veterans: risk of infection, hospitalization, Ventilation, and mortality. Hepatology 2021;74(1):322–35.
37. Marjot T, Moon AM, Cook JA, et al. Outcomes following SARS-CoV-2 infection in patients with chronic liver disease: an international registry study. J Hepatol 2021; 74(3):567–77.
38. Ge J, Pletcher MJ, Lai JC, et al. Outcomes of SARS-CoV-2 infection in patients with chronic liver disease and cirrhosis: a national COVID cohort Collaborative study. Gastroenterology 2021;161(5):1487–501.e5.
39. Bajaj JS, Garcia-Tsao G, Wong F, et al. Cirrhosis is associated with high mortality and readmissions over 90 Days Regardless of COVID-19: a multicenter cohort. Liver Transpl 2021;27(9):1343–7.
40. Global hepatitis report 2017. Geneva: World Health Organization. Available at: cdc.gov/vaccines/adults/rec-vac/health-conditions/liver-disease.html. Accessed April 20, 2022.
41. Blach S, Kondili LA, Aghemo A, et al. Impact of COVID-19 on global HCV elimination efforts. J Hepatol 2021;74(1):31–6.
42. Yip TC, Wong VW, Lui GC, et al. Current and Past infections of HBV do not increase mortality in patients with COVID-19. Hepatology 2021;74(4):1750–65.
43. Ji D, Qin E, Xu J, et al. Non-alcoholic fatty liver diseases in patients with COVID-19: a retrospective study. J Hepatol 2020;73(2):451–3.
44. Sachdeva S, Khandait H, Kopel J, et al. NAFLD and COVID-19: a Pooled analysis. SN Compr Clin Med 2020;2(12):2726–9.
45. Marjot T, Buescher G, Sebode M, et al. SARS-CoV-2 infection in patients with autoimmune hepatitis. J Hepatol 2021;74(6):1335–43.
46. Efe C, Dhanasekaran R, Lammert C, et al. Outcome of COVID-19 in patients with autoimmune hepatitis: an international multicenter study. Hepatology 2021;73(6): 2099–109.
47. Colmenero J, Rodríguez-Perálvarez M, Salcedo M, et al. Epidemiological pattern, incidence, and outcomes of COVID-19 in liver transplant patients. J Hepatol 2021;74(1):148–55.
48. Ravanan R, Callaghan CJ, Mumford L, et al. SARS-CoV-2 infection and early mortality of waitlisted and solid organ transplant recipients in England: a national cohort study. Am J Transplant 2020;20(11):3008–18.
49. Webb GJ, Marjot T, Cook JA, et al. Outcomes following SARS-CoV-2 infection in liver transplant recipients: an international registry study. Lancet Gastroenterol Hepatol 2020;5(11):1008–16.
50. Pereira MR, Mohan S, Cohen DJ, et al. COVID-19 in solid organ transplant recipients: initial report from the US epicenter. Am J Transplant 2020;20(7):1800–8.
51. Rabiee A, Sadowski B, Adeniji N, et al. Liver injury in liver transplant recipients with coronavirus disease 2019 (COVID-19): U.S. Multicenter Experience. Hepatology 2020;72(6):1900–11.

52. Webb GJ, Moon AM, Barnes E, et al. Determining risk factors for mortality in liver transplant patients with COVID-19. Lancet Gastroenterol Hepatol 2020;5(7): 643–4.

53. D'Antiga L. Coronaviruses and immunosuppressed patients: the facts during the Third Epidemic. Liver Transpl 2020;26(6):832–4.

54. Del Valle DM, Kim-Schulze S, Huang HH, et al. An inflammatory cytokine signature predicts COVID-19 severity and survival. Nat Med 2020;26(10):1636–43.

55. Horby P, Lim WS, Emberson JR, et al. Dexamethasone in hospitalized patients with covid-19. N Engl J Med 2021;384(8):693–704.

56. Gerussi A, Rigamonti C, Elia C, et al. Coronavirus Disease 2019 (COVID-19) in autoimmune hepatitis: a lesson from immunosuppressed patients. Hepatol Commun 2020. https://doi.org/10.1002/hep4.1557.

57. Reddy KR, Beavers KL, Hammond SP, et al. American Gastroenterological Association Institute guideline on the prevention and treatment of hepatitis B virus reactivation during immunosuppressive drug therapy. Gastroenterology 2015; 148(1):215–9.

58. Chen LF, Mo YQ, Jing J, et al. Short-course tocilizumab increases risk of hepatitis B virus reactivation in patients with rheumatoid arthritis: a prospective clinical observation. Int J Rheum Dis 2017;20(7):859–69.

59. Fix OK, Serper M. Telemedicine and Telehepatology during the COVID-19 pandemic. Clin Liver Dis (Hoboken) 2020;15(5):187–90.

60. Mann DM, Chen J, Chunara R, et al. COVID-19 transforms health care through telemedicine: evidence from the field. J Am Med Inform Assoc 2020;27(7): 1132–5.

61. Serper M, Cubell AW, Deleener ME, et al. Telemedicine in liver disease and beyond: can the COVID-19 Crisis lead to action? Hepatology 2020;72(2):723–8.

62. Wegermann K, Wilder JM, Parish A, et al. Racial and socioeconomic disparities in Utilization of Telehealth in patients with liver disease during COVID-19. Dig Dis Sci 2022;67(1):93–9.

63. Fix O, Kaul D, et al. AASLD expert panel consensus statement: vaccines to prevent COVID-19 in patient with liver disease . https://aasld.org/VaccineDocument.

64. Fix OK, Blumberg EA, Chang KM, et al. American association for the study of liver diseases expert panel consensus statement: vaccines to prevent coronavirus disease 2019 infection in patients with liver disease. Hepatology 2021;74(2): 1049–64.

65. Polack FP, Thomas SJ, Kitchin N, et al. Safety and efficacy of the BNT162b2 mRNA covid-19 vaccine. N Engl J Med 2020;383(27):2603–15.

66. Baden LR, El Sahly HM, Essink B, et al. Efficacy and safety of the mRNA-1273 SARS-CoV-2 vaccine. N Engl J Med 2021;384(5):403–16.

67. McCashland TM, Preheim LC, Gentry MJ. Pneumococcal vaccine response in cirrhosis and liver transplantation. J Infect Dis 2000;181(2):757–60.

68. Aggeletopoulou I, Davoulou P, Konstantakis C, et al. Response to hepatitis B vaccination in patients with liver cirrhosis. Rev Med Virol 2017;27(6). https://doi.org/10.1002/rmv.1942.

69. John BV, Deng Y, Scheinberg A, et al. Association of BNT162b2 mRNA and mRNA-1273 vaccines with COVID-19 infection and hospitalization among patients with cirrhosis. JAMA Intern Med 2021;181(10):1306–14.

70. Chong PP, Avery RK. A Comprehensive review of immunization Practices in solid organ transplant and Hematopoietic Stem cell transplant recipients. Clin Ther 2017;39(8):1581–98.

71. Caballero-Marcos A, Salcedo M, Alonso-Fernández R, et al. Changes in humoral immune response after SARS-CoV-2 infection in liver transplant recipients compared with immunocompetent patients. Am J Transpl 2021;21(8):2876–84.

72. Rabinowich L, Grupper A, Baruch R, et al. Low immunogenicity to SARS-CoV-2 vaccination among liver transplant recipients. J Hepatol 2021;75(2):435–8.

73. Kamar N, Abravanel F, Marion O, et al. Three doses of an mRNA covid-19 vaccine in solid-organ transplant recipients. N Engl J Med 2021;385(7):661–2.

74. Hall VG, Ferreira VH, Ku T, et al. Randomized trial of a Third dose of mRNA-1273 vaccine in transplant recipients. N Engl J Med 2021;385(13):1244–6.

75. Ruether DF, Schaub GM, Duengelhoef PM, et al. SARS-CoV2-specific humoral and T-cell immune response after second vaccination in liver cirrhosis and transplant patients. Clin Gastroenterol Hepatol 2022;20(1):162–72.e9.

76. Kates OS, Stohs EJ, Pergam SA, et al. The limits of refusal: an ethical review of solid organ transplantation and vaccine hesitancy. Am J Transpl 2021;21(8):2637–45.

77. Lee ARYB, Wong SY, Chai LYA, et al. Efficacy of covid-19 vaccines in immuno-compromised patients: systematic review and meta-analysis. BMJ 2022;376:e068632.

78. CDC. COVID-19 Vaccines for moderately or severely immunocompromised people. https://www.cdc.gov/coronavirus/2019-ncov/vaccines/recommendations/immuno.html. Accessed April 14, 2022.

79. Bril F, Fettig DM. Reply to: "Comment on "Autoimmune hepatitis developing after coronavirus disease 2019 (COVID-19) vaccine: Causality or casualty? J Hepatol 2021;75(4):996–7.

80. McShane C, Kiat C, Rigby J, et al. The mRNA COVID-19 vaccine - a rare trigger of autoimmune hepatitis? J Hepatol 2021;75(5):1252–4.

81. Rocco A, Sgamato C, Compare D, et al. Autoimmune hepatitis following SARS-CoV-2 vaccine: may not be a casuality. J Hepatol 2021;75(3):728–9.

82. Cow KW, Pham NV, Ibrahim BM. Autoimmune hepatitis-like syndrome following COVID-19 vaccination: a systemic review of the literature. Dig Dis Sci 2022.

83. Shroff H, Satapathy SK, Crawford JM, et al. Liver injury following SARS-CoV-2 vaccination: a multicenter case series. J Hepatol 2022;76(1):211–4.

84. Nepogodiev D, Simoes J, Li E, et al. Timing of surgery following SARS-CoV-2 infection: an international prospective cohort study. Anaesthesia 2021;76(6):748–58.

85. Kaul DR, Vece G, Blumberg E, et al. Ten years of donor-derived disease: a report of the disease transmission advisory committee. Am J Transplan 2021;21(2):689–702.

86. Kaul DR, Valesano AL, Petrie JG, et al. Donor to recipient transmission of SARS-CoV-2 by lung transplantation despite negative donor upper respiratory tract testing. Am J Transpl 2021;21(8):2885–9.

87. Kulkarni AV, Parthasarathy K, Kumar P, et al. Early liver transplantation after COVID-19 infection: the first report. Am J Transplant 2021;21(6):2279–84.

88. Koval CE, Poggio ED, Lin YC, et al. Early success transplanting kidneys from donors with new SARS-CoV-2 RNA positivity: a report of 10 cases. Am J Transpl 2021;21(11):3743–9.

89. Sigler R, Shah M, Schnickel G, et al. Successful heart and kidney transplantation from a deceased donor with PCR positive COVID-19. Transpl Infect Dis 2021;23(5):e13707.

90. de la Villa S, Valerio M, Salcedo M, et al. Heart and liver transplant recipients from donor with positive SARS-CoV-2 RT-PCR at time of transplantation. Transpl Infect Dis 2021;23(5):e13664.
91. Meshram HS, Kute VB, Patel H, et al. A case report of successful kidney transplantation from a deceased donor with terminal COVID-19-related lung damage: Ongoing dilemma between discarding and accepting organs in COVID-19 era. Transpl Infect Dis 2021;23(5):e13683.
92. Cariani L, Orena BS, Ambrogi F, et al. Time length of Negativization and cycle threshold Values in 182 health care Workers with covid-19 in milan, Italy: an Observational cohort study. Int J Environ Res Public Health 2020;(15):17. https://doi.org/10.3390/ijerph17155313.
93. Fix OK, Hameed B, Fontana RJ, et al. Clinical best Practice Advice for hepatology and liver transplant providers during the COVID-19 pandemic: AASLD expert panel consensus statement. Hepatology 2020;72(1):287–304.
94. Belli LS, Fondevila C, Cortesi PA, et al. Protective role of Tacrolimus, Deleterious role of age and comorbidities in liver transplant recipients with covid-19: results from the ELITA/ELTR Multi-center European study. Gastroenterology 2021; 160(4):1151–63.e3.
95. Hammond J, Leister-Tebbe H, Gardner A, et al. Oral nirmatrelvir for high-risk, Nonhospitalized adults with covid-19. N Engl J Med 2022;386(15):1397–408.
96. Coronavirus NIH. Disease 2019 (COVID-19) treatment guidelines. Available at: http://www.covid19treatmentguidelines.nih.gov. Accessed April 23, 2022.

Pruritus in Chronic Liver Disease

Ranya Selim, MD[a],*, Joseph Ahn, MD[b]

KEYWORDS

- Pruritus • Liver disease • Cholestasis

KEY POINTS

- Pruritus can often be a symptom of chronic liver disease.
- Cholestyramine is the first-line treatment; if this fails, alternative medical therapy, phototherapy, plasmapheresis, dialysis, and biliary diversion can be considered.
- Severe refractory pruritus can be an indication for liver transplantation.

INTRODUCTION

Pruritus describes the sensation of discomfort or irritation that provokes a need to scratch, also known more colloquially as "itching." Pruritus associated with liver disease has been described as early as 200 BC.[1] Some of the classic chronic liver diseases that are especially associated with pruritus include primary biliary cirrhosis (occurring in many of these patients along their disease course), cholestasis of pregnancy, and primary sclerosing cholangitis. Pruritus can also less commonly be associated with viral hepatitis, obstructive jaundice, and drug-induced liver injury with cholestasis.[2]

Pruritus in chronic liver disease often begins in the palms and soles, subsequently becoming generalized. It tends to be intermittent, chronic, and worse in the evening and at warmer temperatures. Occasionally, pruritus can be severe enough to significantly affect quality of life. Although the severity of pruritus does not necessarily relate to the prognosis of the underlying liver disease, severe and refractory pruritus may be an indication for orthotopic liver transplantation.[2]

Much is still being discovered about the exact pathophysiology of pruritus or the precise mechanism of action of certain therapies.[1,2] This review summarizes the current literature regarding pruritus in patients with chronic liver disease.

[a] Division of Gastroenterology and Hepatology, Henry Ford Health System, 2799 W Grand Boulevard, Detroit, MI 48202, USA; [b] Division of Gastroenterology and Hepatology, Oregon Health and Science University, 3181 Southwest Sam Jackson, Portland, OR 97239, USA
* Corresponding author.
E-mail address: ranyaselim@gmail.com

Clin Liver Dis 27 (2023) 47–55
https://doi.org/10.1016/j.cld.2022.08.011
1089-3261/23/© 2022 Elsevier Inc. All rights reserved.

EPIDEMIOLOGY

The prevalence of pruritus in chronic liver disease varies by underlying cause of liver disease and has not been confirmed in large-scale studies. Pruritus is reported in up to 70% of patients with primary biliary cholangitis, often preceding the diagnosis. Studies have demonstrated that 2.5% to 30% of patients with hepatitis C and 8% of patients with hepatitis B were found to have pruritus.[3–5] Intrahepatic cholestasis of pregnancy classically presents with pruritus in pregnancy due to increase serum bile acids. The prevalence of pruritus in autoimmune hepatitis, alcoholic liver disease, and nonalcoholic fatty liver disease has not been clearly established.[5] Benign causes of obstructive jaundice tend to be associated with a lower rate of pruritus as compared with malignant causes (16% vs 45%, respectively).[2]

PATHOPHYSIOLOGY/CAUSE

There are several proposed mechanisms of pruritus in liver disease.

One theory suggests that pruritus can be caused by the accumulation of bile salts, especially in cholestatic conditions, which are thought to trigger mast cell degranulation.[6] It is notable, however, that not all patients with elevated bile acids were found to develop pruritus, and thus bile acids are not believed to be solely responsible for pruritic symptoms. It has been proposed that bile acids may cause to hepatocyte toxicity, leading to spillage of hepatocyte contents that are potentially pruritogenic.[7]

More recently, lysophosphatidic acid and autotaxin have additionally been suggested to be involved in the development of itching in cholestatic patients.[8,9] Autotaxin is an enzyme that is involved in the production of lysophosphatidic acid, a phospholipid that is involved in multiple different pathways. Although the exact mechanism leading to pruritus has not been determined, autotaxin levels have been shown to correlate to the degree of itching.[10]

Another suggested mechanism is the production of endogenous opioids and activation of their receptors leading to pruritus. It is thought that activation of μ-opioid receptors may illicit pruritus by reducing pain signaling; this is the basis of utilization of μ-opioid receptor antagonists with some efficacy in these patients, which is discussed further later.[2]

It is important to note, however, that the aforementioned mechanisms have not been confirmed, and the relationship between these proposed factors and pruritus is as of yet unclear.[11]

RISK FACTORS

It is not entirely clear what risk factors affect the severity of pruritus. However, few factors have been identified that may increase the risk of developing pruritus. Advanced age is often associated with the development of xerosis, which can promote itching. Alternatively, this population can develop various dermatitides associated with itching as well. Diabetes has also been reported to be associated with a higher risk of pruritus.[5] One retrospective data suggested that women were more likely to report pruritus due to a variety of systemic illnesses as compared with men.[12] Finally, race/ethnicity is thought to potentially play a role in the development of pruritus, given the varying prevalence among different populations, although further studies are needed to identify why these differences exist.[13,14] Oeda and colleagues assessed more than 1600 patients with chronic liver disease and determined that active hepatitis B, primary biliary cholangitis, aspartate aminotransferase greater than or equal to 60 U/L, and diabetes were independent risk factors for pruritus.[5]

EVALUATION

The first step in the evaluation of the cause of pruritus is to determine whether a rash, which would suggest a dermatologic disorder, is present. If this is ruled out, alternative disorders to consider include systemic (both hepatic and extrahepatic), neurologic, and psychogenic disorders. Localized pruritus suggests either a neurologic or psychogenic disorder.[15]

  A detailed history should be obtained including presence of risk factors for liver disease, comorbidities, constitutional symptoms, and medication/substance use. Patient questionnaires can be used at initial evaluation and during treatment to determine the impact of pruritus and response to therapy. Various standardized scales, such as the Numerical Rating Scale, Dermatology Life Quality Index, and 5D Itch Scale, have been used in clinical trials to objectively quantify the severity of pruritus. These scales measure the characteristics of pruritus such as distribution and intensity, with some assessing for associated conditions such as anxiety, depression, and insomnia, as well as overall quality of life.[34]

  Physical examination should include an evaluation for stigmata of chronic liver diseases such as palmar erythema, spider angiomata, and gynecomastia. Laboratory evaluation may include a liver profile, coagulation profile, viral serologies, autoimmune serologies, and bile salts, depending on the clinical history. If biliary obstruction is suspected, ultrasound and/or cross-sectional imaging should be obtained.[15] **Fig. 1** outlines a clinical approach to patients with pruritus.

MANAGEMENT STRATEGIES

An initial approach to symptomatic relief may involve a trial of moisturizers or cooling ointments. Topical antihistamines may be attempted but have generally been found to be ineffective. If topical therapies do not provide relief, there are several potential mechanisms of relieving symptoms. These include removal and alteration of metabolism of pruritogenic substances, modulating itch signaling, or biliary drainage in the case of obstruction.

Medication Regimens

Antihistamines, such as hydroxyzine and diphenhydramine, are often used as initial therapy for pruritus given their relative safety and availability. An additional benefit of antihistamines (particularly H1 antihistamines) is their sedative effect, which may be helpful in those with nocturnal symptoms. Despite this, there are limited efficacy data regarding these, and alternative or complimentary agents often need to be used.[33]

  Ursodiol is a bile acid that has been shown to be ineffective in relieving pruritus in primary sclerosing cholangitis and primary biliary cirrhosis. However, ursodiol has been found to alleviate pruritus in intrahepatic cholestasis of pregnancy, and thus it is only indicated for this condition. It is typically administered at a dose of 10 to 15 mg/kg/d in 2 to 3 divided doses.[16,17]

  Cholestyramine is a bile salt resin that has been shown to be effective in relieving cholestatic pruritus and is the typical first-line treatment. It is generally well tolerated, although with potential side effects including gastrointestinal upset, constipation, and rarely fat malabsorption.[18,19] Dosing is typically 4 g 1 to 2 times a day, up to 16 g/d in divided doses. Importantly, cholestyramine can bind other medications, so other drugs need to be administered 1 hour before or at least 4 to 6 hours following cholestyramine dose.[20]

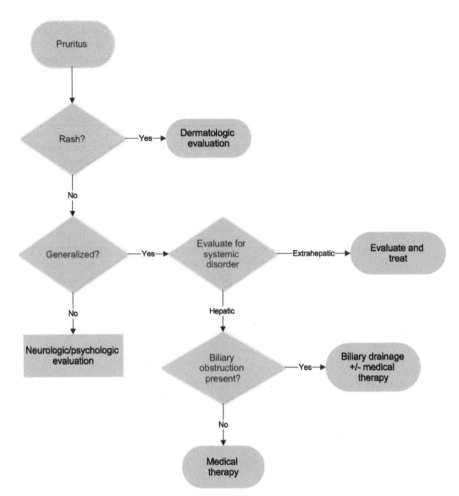

Fig. 1. Diagnostic approach to pruritus.

Rifampicin was shown to reduce autotaxin expression and ameliorate pruritus, particularly in those with refractory itching and malignant cholestasis.[21,22] Rifampicin has been safely used in patients with cholestatic pruritus; however, there is a risk hepatotoxicity in up to 13% of patients when used for prolonged periods. Other potential side effects include hemolytic anemia, renal failure, and thrombocytopenia; therefore, complete blood counts and liver function tests should be monitored during therapy. Dosing is typically 150 to 300 mg twice daily.[23]

Naloxone and naltrexone are μ-opioid receptor antagonists that have been shown to be effective in treating cholestatic pruritus in prospective trials. These are contraindicated in patients with acute liver injury or failure and should be avoided in patients on narcotics. Naltrexone is typically administered at a dose of 25 to 50 mg daily. Nalfurafine is a κ-opioid agonist that is primarily metabolized by cytochrome P450, producing an inactive metabolite. In a randomized trial conducted in 2017, 109 patients were treated with 5 μg nalfurafine, 105 patients were treated with 2.5 μg nalfurafine, and 103 patients received placebo. Patients treated with nalfurafine had significantly greater improvement in their pruritus scores as compared with those who received placebo.

In addition, no significant adverse events were experienced with either dose of nalfurafine.[24,25]

Sertraline has been shown to be well tolerated with modest reduction in pruritic symptoms. This drug should be used with caution in patients with advanced liver disease due to primary liver metabolism.[26] Sertraline should also be avoided within 14 days of administration of monoamine oxidase and should not be co-administered with disulfiram.[27]

Alternative Therapies

Patients who are refractory to or poor candidates for the aforementioned agents may attempt alternative experimental therapies. The data regarding these modalities are limited to case reports and case series. Thus the efficacy of these methods has not yet been validated.

Experimental drug therapies for pruritus include thalidomide, ondansetron, and phenobarbital. Thalidomide is an immunomodulator with potential antipruritic effects, thought to be secondary to a central depressant effect.[28] Ondansetron is a serotonin receptor antagonist that is primarily used as an antiemetic. Data regarding its use for pruritus in patients with liver disease are mixed and evidence supporting its use is mostly anecdotal. Phenobarbital is primarily an anticonvulsant that has been attempted for the management of refractory pruritus. Data regarding phenobarbital use for liver disease–related pruritus has not shown clear benefit.[1]

Other therapies include plasmapheresis, ultraviolet (UV) phototherapy, albumin dialysis, and nasobiliary drainage. Given the more invasive nature of some of these modalities, they tend to be considered mainly when patients have failed the aforementioned more traditional therapies.

Some studies have shown improvement in pruritic symptoms with plasmapheresis. The exact mechanism by which plasmapheresis mitigates pruritus is not clear, although it has been suggested that it may reduce autotaxin activity. Although plasmapheresis is not used routinely for pruritis, it can be considered for refractory cases when available, particularly as a bridge to definitive therapy.[29]

UV phototherapy has shown success limited to case reports. It has been suggested that this may improve pruritus through interaction with itch receptors at the dermoepidermal junction or alternatively by inactivating pruritogens in the skin. Another well-established effect of UV therapy is excretion of bile acids in urine. Available data mainly include case reports and observational studies on dermatology. However, there is a lack of data regarding its use in cholestatic pruritus, and thus phototherapy has not been adopted as standard of care at this time.[30]

Nasobiliary drainage involves endoscopically placing a nasobiliary catheter into the common bile duct, the distal end of which is subsequently passed through the nasal canal and connected to an external bag. Data regarding nasobiliary damage are limited to few single-center studies but has generally shown positive results in terms of symptom relief as well as improvement in alkaline phosphatase and bilirubin levels.[31]

Albumin dialysis involves a hemofiltration system that uses albumin-enriched dialysate to remove pruritogenic substances from blood. Small studies involving the use of albumin dialysis showed sustained relief of pruritus as well as a decline in serum bile acids, with minimal side effects.[32]

Surgical Therapy

Partial biliary diversion interrupts enterohepatic circulation of bile salts, bypassing terminal ileal resorption, leading to a reduction of the bile acid pool and thereby

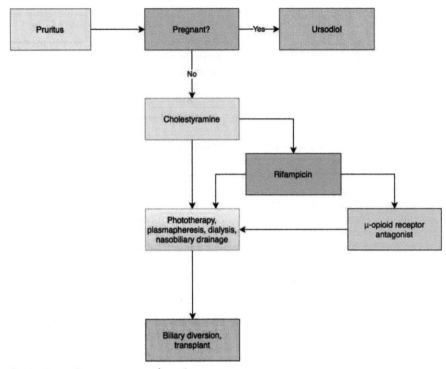

Fig. 2. General management of pruritus.

improving pruritus. In the past, external biliary diversion was performed. More recently, however, partial internal biliary diversion has been used, which involves diverting bile from the gallbladder to the colon, bypassing the terminal ileum. However, data regarding biliary diversion have been quite limited, mainly in children with progressive familial intrahepatic cholestasis. In this population, normalization of liver biochemistries, decrease in bile acids, and relief of pruritus has been demonstrated. Ileal exclusion is an alternative to biliary diversion that has been shown to result in symptomatic relief, although associated with recurrence of symptoms in half of the patients.[30]

Occasionally pruritus can be severe enough to cause fatigue, depression, and suicidality. Orthotopic liver transplantation can be considered as a last resort for refractory pruritus associated with chronic liver disease significantly affecting quality of life, even in the absence of liver failure. This treatment should be reserved for patients who have failed an adequate trial of medical (and perhaps some experimental) therapies noted earlier.[2] **Fig. 2** outlines a management approach to pruritus.

SUMMARY

Pruritus associated with chronic liver disease occurs due to complex, incompletely understood pathophysiology. Occasionally this can be disturbing enough to patients to affect their quality of life, and in these patients more invasive therapies including liver transplantation may need to be considered if pruritus is refractory to medical therapy. Further studies are needed to elucidate the complete pathophysiology of pruritus in chronic liver disease, which would aid in the development of additional effective therapies for this condition.

DISCLOSURE

The authors have nothing to disclose.

CLINICS CARE POINTS

- Pruritus associated with chronic liver disease is most commonly associated with cholestatic liver disease but can be seen associated with other chronic liver diseases as well.
- Liver disease–associated pruritus tends to begin with an acral distribution, subsequently becoming generalized.
- The presence of a rash with localized pruritus suggests a dermatologic cause of pruritus.
- Localized pruritus in the absence of a rash suggests a neurologic or psychogenic cause of pruritus.
- Ursodiol, although helpful in improving biochemical parameters in primary biliary cholangitis, is not effective in relieving pruritus except for patients with intrahepatic cholestasis of pregnancy.
- Cholestyramine is most often the first-line therapy for pruritus in liver disease. Medications should be administered 1 hour before or at least 4 to 6 hours following cholestyramine dose.
- Complete blood counts and liver function tests should be monitored while on rifampicin therapy.
- μ-Opioid receptor antagonists should be avoided in patients on opioids.
- Plasmapheresis, phototherapy, albumin dialysis, and nasobiliary drainage can be considered in patients with pruritus refractory to medical therapy.
- Liver transplantation can be considered in select patients with refractory pruritus.

REFERENCES

1. Bhalerao A, Mannu GS. Management of pruritus in chronic liver disease. Dermatol Res Pract 2015;2015:295891. https://doi.org/10.1155/2015/295891.
2. Tajiri K, Shimizu Y. Recent advances in the management of pruritus in chronic liver diseases. World J Gastroenterol 2017;23(19):3418–26.
3. Dega H, Francès C, Dupin N, et al. Prurit et virus de l'hépatite C. Le Groupe Multivirc [Pruritus and the hepatitis C virus. The MULTIVIRC Unit]. Ann Dermatol Venereol 1998;125(1):9–12. French. PMID: 9747198.
4. Montagnese S, Nsemi LM, Cazzagon N, et al. Sleep-Wake profiles in patients with primary biliary cirrhosis. Liver Int 2013;33(2):203–9. Epub 2012 Nov 22. PMID: 23173839.
5. Oeda S, Takahashi H, Yoshida H, et al. Prevalence of pruritus in patients with chronic liver disease: a multicenter study. Hepatol Res 2018;48:E252–62. https://doi.org/10.1111/hepr.12978.
6. Langedijk JAGM, Beuers UH, Oude Elferink RPJ. Cholestasis-associated pruritus and its pruritogens. Front Med (Lausanne) 2021;8:639674. https://doi.org/10.3389/fmed.2021.639674.
7. Ghent CN. Pruritus of cholestasis is related to effects of bile salts on the liver, not the skin. Am J Gastroenterol 1987;82(2):117–8. PMID: 3812415.
8. Kittaka H, Uchida K, Fukuta N, et al. Lysophosphatidic acid-induced itch is mediated by signalling of LPA. J Physiol 2017;595(8):2681–98.

9. Kremer AE, et al. Lysophosphatidic acid is a potential mediator of cholestatic pruritus. Gastroenterology 2010;139(3):1008–18.

10. Wunsch E, Krawczyk M, Milkiewicz M, et al. Serum autotaxin is a Marker of the severity of liver injury and overall Survival in patients with cholestatic liver diseases. Sci Rep 2016;6:30847. https://doi.org/10.1038/srep30847.

11. Jones EA, Bergasa NV. The pruritus of cholestasis: from bile acids to opiate agonists. Hepatology 1990;11(5):884–7.

12. Beuers U, Kremer AE, Bolier R, et al. Pruritus in cholestasis: Facts and fiction. Hepatology 2014;60:399–407.

13. Peters MG, Di Bisceglie AM, Kowdley KV, et al. Differences between Caucasian, African American, and Hispanic patients with primary biliary cirrhosis in the United States. Hepatology 2007;46:769–75.

14. Abedin P, Weaver JB, Egginton E. Intrahepatic cholestasis of pregnancy: prevalence and ethnic distribution. Ethn Health 1999;4(1–2):35–7.

15. Yosipovitch G, Bernhard JD. Clinical practice. Chronic pruritus. N Engl J Med 2013;368(17):1625–34.

16. Zein CO, Lindor KD. Latest and emerging therapies for primary biliary cirrhosis and primary sclerosing cholangitis. Curr Gastroenterol Rep 2010;12(1):13–22.

17. Glantz A, Reilly S-J, Benthin L, et al. Intrahepatic cholestasis of pregnancy: amelioration of pruritus by UDCA is associated with decreased progesterone disulphates in urine. Hepatology 2008;47(2):544–51.

18. di Padova C, Tritapepe R, Rovagnati P, et al. Double-blind placebo-controlled clinical trial of microporous cholestyramine in the treatment of intra- and extrahepatic cholestasis: relationship between itching and serum bile acids. Methods Findings Exp Clin Pharmacol 1984;6(12):773–6.

19. Duncan JS, Kennedy HJ, Triger DR. Treatment of pruritus due to chronic obstructive liver disease. Br Med J 1984;288(6436):22.

20. Jacobson TA, Armani A, McKenney JM, et al. Safety considerations with gastrointestinally active lipid-lowering drugs. Am J Cardiol 2007;99(6A):47C–55C.

21. Levy C, Lindor KD. Current management of primary biliary cirrhosis and primary sclerosing cholangitis. J Hepatol 2003;38(supplement 1):S24–37.

22. Price TJ, Patterson WK, Olver IN. Rifampicin as treatment for pruritus in malignant cholestasis. Support Care Cancer 1998;6(6):533–5.

23. Prince MI, Burt AD, Jones DEJ. Hepatitis and liver dysfunction with rifampicin therapy for pruritus in primary biliary cirrhosis. Gut 2002;50(3):436–9.

24. Bergasa NV, Ailing DW, Talbot TL, et al. Effects of naloxone infusions in patients with the pruritus of cholestasis: a double-blind, randomized, controlled trial. Ann Intern Med 1995;123(3):161–7.

25. Phan NQ, Bernhard JD, Luger TA, et al. Antipruritic treatment with systemic μ-opioid receptor antagonists: a review. J Am Acad Dermatol 2010;63(4):680–8.

26. Mayo MJ, Handem I, Saldana S, et al. Sertraline as a first-line treatment for cholestatic pruritus. Hepatology 2007;45(3):666–74.

27. Sola CL, Bostwick JM, Hart DA, et al. Anticipating potential linezolid-SSRI interactions in the general hospital setting: an MAOI in disguise. Mayo Clin Proc 2006 Mar;81(3):330–4.

28. Adams F. The extant works of aretaeus, the cappadocian. London, UK: Sydenham Society; 1865.

29. Heerkens M, Dedden S, Scheepers H, et al. Effect of plasmapheresis on cholestatic pruritus and autotaxin Activity during pregnancy. Hepatology 2019;69:2707–10.

30. Pinheiro NC, Marinho RT, Ramalho F, et al. Refractory pruritus in primary biliary cirrhosis. BMJ Case Rep 2013;2013. https://doi.org/10.1136/bcr-2013-200634. bcr2013200634.
31. Hegade VS, Krawczyk M, Kremer AE, et al. The safety and efficacy of nasobiliary drainage in the treatment of refractory cholestatic pruritus: a multicentre European study. Aliment Pharmacol Ther 2016;43:294–302.
32. Carpentier B, Gautier A, Legallais C. Artificial and bioartificial liver devices: present and future. Gut 2009 Dec;58(12):1690–702.
33. Pinheiro NC, Marinho RT, Ramalho F, et al. Refractory pruritus in primary biliary cirrhosis. BMJ Case Rep 2013;2013. bcr2013200634.
34. Ständer S, Augustin M, Reich A, Ständer S, Augustin M, Reich A,. International Forum for the Study of Itch Special Interest Group Scoring Itch in Clinical Trials. Pruritus assessment in clinical trials: consensus recommendations from the International Forum for the Study of Itch (IFSI) Special Interest Group Scoring Itch in Clinical Trials. Acta Derm Venereol 2013;93(5):509–14.

Renal Insufficiency in Patients with Cirrhosis

Caroline L. Matchett, MD[a], Douglas A. Simonetto, MD[b], Patrick S. Kamath, MD[b],*

KEYWORDS

- Acute kidney injury • Renal insufficiency • Cirrhosis • Hepatorenal syndrome
- International ascites club

KEY POINTS

- Acute kidney injury (AKI), including hepatorenal syndrome, is a common complication in patients with cirrhosis and is associated with high morbidity and mortality.
- The International Club of Ascites has defined AKI in cirrhosis based predominantly on the percentage of serum creatinine increase from the baseline.
- The use of urinary biomarkers of tubular damage may aid in the differential diagnosis of AKI in cirrhosis.
- Advances in our understanding of the pathophysiology of AKI and cirrhosis have led to changes in our approach to renal insufficiency in patients with cirrhosis.

INTRODUCTION

Acute kidney injury (AKI) is a frequent complication in patients hospitalized with complications of cirrhosis and is associated with high morbidity and mortality. Prerenal azotemia, hepatorenal syndrome (HRS)–AKI and acute tubular necrosis (ATN) represent the most common etiologies of AKI in patients with advanced liver disease. Differentiating these conditions may be challenging, but is required due to the differences in the treatment of each etiology. HRS–AKI is characterized by functional circulatory changes that ultimately lead to impairment in kidney function. There have been recent advances in defining this clinical entity and addressing optimal management. This review highlights the contemporary criteria, pathophysiology, diagnosis, and management of renal failure and HRS in patients with cirrhosis.

EPIDEMIOLOGY AND DEFINITIONS

The reported incidence of AKI ranges from 20% to 50% in patients with cirrhosis admitted to the hospital.[1–3] The traditional definition of AKI in cirrhosis was based

[a] Internal Medicine Residency Program, Department of Medicine, Mayo Clinic, 200 1st Street Southwest, Rochester, 55902 MN, USA; [b] Division of Gastroenterology and Hepatology, Department of Medicine, Mayo Clinic, 200 1st Street Southwest, Rochester, 55902 MN, USA
* Corresponding author.
E-mail address: kamath.patrick@mayo.edu

Clin Liver Dis 27 (2023) 57–70
https://doi.org/10.1016/j.cld.2022.08.010
1089-3261/23/© 2022 Elsevier Inc. All rights reserved.

on an increased serum creatinine value of greater than 1.5 mg/dl.[4] This definition had limitations in that it relied on a fixed threshold that did not account for dynamic changes in serum creatinine that are essential in distinguishing acute from chronic renal insufficiency.[5]

The definition of AKI has gone through many updates over the last 2 decades as enumerated in **Table 1**. In 2004, the Consensus Conference of the Acute Dialysis Quality Initiative Group defined the risk, injury, failure, loss, and end-stage kidney disease (RIFLE) classification, which was based on changes in serum creatinine or glomerular filtration rate (GFR) and urine output.[6] Three years later (2007) this classification was refined by the Acute Kidney Injury Network (AKIN) to include the full spectrum of acute renal injury and adjusted the definition of AKI to include an absolute increase in baseline serum creatinine of 0.3 mg/dL within 48 hours.[7] In 2012, the Kidney Disease Improving Global Outcome (KDIGO) further refined the RIFLE and AKIN criteria for defining AKI as an increase in serum creatinine by at least 0.3 mg/dL within 48 hours, an increase in serum creatinine to at least 1.5 times the baseline within the last 7 days, or urine volume less than 0.5 mL/kg/h for 6 hours.[8]

The International Club of Ascites (ICA) modified the definition of AKI with a prognostic significance for cirrhosis and formed the ICA–AKI criteria (**Box 1**).[9] This classification system is based predominately on the percentage of serum creatinine increase from the baseline. The ICA also eliminated urine output from the revised definition of AKI, owing to the expected reduced urine output in patients with cirrhosis due to avid sodium retention.

The definition of HRS has also evolved over time. Formerly, HRS was categorized into two major types: type 1, defined by rapid impairment of renal function manifested in less than 2 weeks by doubling of initial serum creatinine to a level greater than 2.5 mg/dL or a 50% reduction of the initial 24 h creatinine clearance to a level lower than 20 mL/min; and type 2, defined by a less rapid course of renal impairment.[4] The changes proposed by the KDIGO guidelines prompted the ICA in 2015 to reclassify the previous HRS type 1 as the acute form of HRS–AKI,[9] and in 2019, HRS type 2 as HRS–NAKI (ie, non-AKI) (**Table 2**).[10] The updated definition of HRS–AKI removed the 2 week interval required for doubling of serum creatinine and the 2.5 mg/dL level cut-off, facilitating earlier diagnosis and treatment. HRS–NAKI is defined by estimated GFR (eGFR) rather than by serum creatinine and divided into HRS–acute kidney disease (HRS–AKD) if the eGFR is less than 60 mL/min/1.73 m² for less than 3 months, and HRS–chronic kidney disease (HRS–CKD) if the eGFR is less than this for greater than 3 months.[11]

PATHOPHYSIOLOGY OF HEPATORENAL SYNDROME

HRS refers to renal dysfunction specific to patients with liver disease and has unique pathophysiology.[12] There has been notable evolution in our understanding of the pathophysiologic mechanisms of HRS in the last several decades.

The *arterial vasodilation theory* has been the leading hypothesis for the development of HRS for the last 20 years. Cirrhosis results in increased intrahepatic vascular resistance associated with overproduction and release of vasodilators (nitric oxide, prostaglandins, endocannabinoids) in the splanchnic and systemic circulation.[13] Splanchnic and systemic vasodilation lead to reduced effective arterial blood volume and systemic arterial hypotension, which in turn lead to a compensatory increase in cardiac output and activation of systemic vasoconstrictor pathways, such as the renin–angiotensin–aldosterone system and the sympathetic nervous system. These mechanisms are typically effective in maintaining circulatory volume in compensated

Table 1
Consensus definitions for acute kidney injury

Criteria	Stage	Definition sCr or GFR Criteria	UOP Criteria
Acute Dialysis Quality Initiative Group -RIFLE criteria in 2004	Stage 1 (risk)	Increased sCr ≥ 1.5 × baseline or GFR decreased > 25%	UOP < .5 mL/kg/h for ≥ 6 h
	Stage 2 (injury)	Increased sCr ≥ 2 × baseline or GFR decreased > 50%	UOP < .5 mL/kg/h for ≥12 h
	Stage 3 (failure)	Increased sCr ≥ 3 × baseline or GFR decreased > 75%	UOP < .3 mL/kg/h for ≥ 24 h
	Loss	Persistent acute renal failure >4 wk	
	End-stage	Complete loss of kidney function > 3 moths	
Acute Kidney Injury Network (AKIN) in 2007	Stage 1	Increased sCr ≥ 1.5 × baseline or ≥ 0.3 mg/dL within 48 h	UOP < .5 mL/kg/h for ≥ 6 h
	Stage 2	Increased sCr ≥ 2 × baseline	UOP < .5 mL/kg/h for ≥ 12 h
	Stage 3	Increased sCr ≥ 3 × baseline	UOP < .3 mL/kg/h for ≥ 24 h or anuria ≥ 12 h
KDIGO in 2012	Stage 1	Increased sCr ≥ 1.5-2 × baseline or ≥ 0.3 mg/dL	UOP < .5 mL/kg/h for ≥ 6-12 h
	Stage 2	Increased sCr ≥ 2-3 × baseline	UOP < .5 mL/kg/h for ≥ 12 h
	Stage 3	Increased sCr ≥ 3 × baseline or sCr ≥ 4.0 mg/dL	UOP < .3 mL/kg/h for 24 h or anuria for ≥ 12 h

Abbreviations: hGFR, glomerular kidney function; RRT, renal replacement therapy; sCr, Serum creatinine; UOP, Urine output.

Box 1
International Club of Ascites stages of acute kidney injury

Stage 1
  Increase in serum creatinine greater than or equal to 0.3 mg/dL (26.5 μmol/L) or increase in serum creatinine less than or equal to 1.5-fold or more to 2-fold from the baseline
    Stage 1a
      Creatinine less than 1.5 mg/dL
    Stage 1b
      Creatinine greater than or equal to 1.5 mg/dL

Stage 2
  Increase in serum creatinine at least 2-fold to 3-fold from the baseline

Stage 3
  Increase in serum creatinine at least threefold from baseline or serum creatinine greater than or equal to 4.0 mg/dL (353.6 μmol/L) with an acute increase of greater than or equal to 0.3 mg/dL (26.5 μmol/L) or the initiation of renal replacement therapy

---

cirrhosis; however, in decompensated cirrhosis, these systems are insufficient, resulting in impaired renal blood flow and consequent functional and ischemic kidney injury.

Systemic inflammation is a more recently described mechanism in the pathophysiology of HRS. Translocation of gut bacteria or bacterial products leads to increased pathogen-associated molecular patterns, such as lipopolysaccharide, flagellin, and nigericin, in the portal circulation. Similarly, hepatocellular injury leads to the release of damage-associated molecular patterns including heat shock protein, double-stranded genomic DNA, and adenosine triphosphate, among others. This proinflammatory response results in increased production of arterial vasodilators and consequent reduction in effective arterial blood volume and systemic vascular resistance leading to renal impairment.[14]

In addition, the hepato-adrenal syndrome may play a role in the development of HRS. Relative adrenal insufficiency is seen in 24% to 49% of patients with decompensated cirrhosis.[15,16] Adrenal insufficiency results in decreased arterial pressure and increased renin and norepinephrine placing these patients at higher risk for the development of HRS–AKI.[16]

Cholemic (bile cast) nephropathy[17] and intra-abdominal hypertension[18] in patients with refractory ascites have also been implicated in the development of HRS.

DIFFERENTIAL DIAGNOSIS

Besides HRS–AKI, other more common causes of renal failure are seen with cirrhosis (ie, hypovolemia, parenchymal disease, nephrotoxicity). Despite the significant overlap, distinguishing the main driver of renal failure in cirrhosis is important for prognostic and therapeutic purposes. Prerenal azotemia and ATN generally confer a better prognosis in cirrhosis, as compared with the markedly dismal prognosis in patients with HRS–AKI.[19]

Differentiating HRS–AKI from ATN remains difficult. The diagnosis of HRS–AKI requires the absence of shock, proteinuria, microhematuria, and normal renal ultrasound.[10] Patients who meet these criteria may still have tubular damage, thus ATN cannot be entirely excluded. Moreover, classical urine biomarkers such as urine sodium and fractional excretion of sodium (FeNa) used for the differential diagnosis of AKI have limitations in patients with cirrhosis. Thus, urine sodium and FeNa are no longer part of the diagnostic criteria for HRS–AKI.

Table 2
Previous and new classifications of hepatorenal syndrome

Old Classification	New Classification	Criteria

HRS type	HRS-AKI	• Increase in sCr ≥ 0.3 mg/dl within 48 h
		OR
		• Increase in sCr ≥ 1.5 times from baseline (sCr value within previous 3 mo, when available, maybe uses baseline, and value closest to presentation should be used)
		• No response to diuretic withdrawal and 2 d fluid challenge with 1 g/kg/d of albumin 20%–25%
		• Cirrhosis with ascites
		• Absence of shock
		• No current or recent use of nephrotoxic drugs (NSAIDs, contrast dye, etc.)
		• No signs of structural kidney injury
		  ○ Absence of proteinuria (>500 mg/d)
		  ○ Absence of hematuria (>50 RBCs per high-power field)
		  ○ Normal findings on renal ultrasound

HRS type 2	HRS–NAKI HRS–AKD HRS–CKD	• eGFR < 60 mL/min per 1.73 m² for < 3 mo in absence of other potential causes of kidney disease • Percentage increase in sCr <50% using last available value of outpatient sCr within 3 mo as baseline value HRS-CKD • eGFR < 60 mL/min per 1.73 m² for ≥ 3 mo in absence of other potential causes of kidney disease

ROLE OF BIOMARKERS

Several novel urinary biomarkers of tubular damage have been investigated to differentiate ATN from HRS–AKI. Tubular proteins released during cell damage (neutrophil gelatinase-associated lipocalin [NGAL]), kidney injury molecule-1, and liver-type fatty acid-binding protein and markers of inflammation (interleukin-18 [IL-18]) are a few of the biomarkers studied for this purpose. Among these, NGAL and IL-18 are the most widely studied and demonstrate the most promising results.

NGAL is a protein expressed by injured kidney tubular epithelia and rises exponentially early during tubular damage.[20] Several studies have demonstrated that urine NGAL has high accuracy in differentiating ATN from HRS–AKI and hypovolemia-induced AKI.[20–22] Urinary NGAL performs best after the 2 days of plasma expansion with albumin that is recommended in the management of AKI. In this setting, the urinary NGAL cut-off value of greater than 220 μg/g of creatinine had the highest diagnostic accuracy for ATN.[21] Studies have also shown that urinary NGAL is an independent predictor of short-term mortality.[20,21] A limitation of NGAL is that levels are also increased in patients with urinary tract infections due to its expression by leukocytes.[23]

IL-18 is a proinflammatory cytokine expressed in the proximal tubule, which is released during tubular injury.[24] Significantly higher IL-18 levels have been observed in patients with cirrhosis and ATN compared with other causes of renal injury. As with NGAL, data also suggest a correlation between IL-18 levels and short-term mortality.[25,26]

RISK FACTORS AND PREVENTION

Predictors of HRS–AKI include hyponatremia, high plasma renin activity, liver size,[13] and severity of ascites.[27,28] The prevalence of HRS–AKI in the absence of identifiable precipitating events is only 1.8%.[28] The most common precipitant of HRS–AKI is large volume paracentesis without albumin administration. Albumin supplementation (6–8 g/L of ascitic fluid removed) post-large volume paracentesis ($\geq$4–5 L) significantly reduces the risk of HRS–AKI and short-term mortality.[29,30] This protective effect is unique to albumin compared with other volume expanders, which may be explained by its antioxidant, anti-inflammatory, endothelial-stabilizing, and endotoxin-inactivation properties.[30–33]

The acute hemodynamic changes associated with infection are another major risk factor for HRS–AKI. Roughly 30% of patients with spontaneous bacterial peritonitis (SBP) developed HRS–AKI.[34] Albumin administration (at a recommended dose of 1.5 g/kg on day 1 and 1 g/kg on day 3) in addition to antibiotic treatment reduces the incidence of SBP-associated HRS–AKI and improves overall survival.[35]

In addition, patients with low ascitic protein fluid (<1.5 mg/dL) associated with liver or kidney dysfunction (Child-Turcotte-Pugh score $\geq$9 with bilirubin $\geq$ 3 mg/dL, or serum creatinine $\geq$1.2 mg/dL, serum sodium $\leq$ 130 mEq/L or blood urea nitrogen $\geq$25) are at increased risk for SBP. Antibiotic prophylaxis prevents the development of SBP and reduces the risk of HRS–AKI and mortality.[35,36]

MANAGEMENT

Early recognition and treatment of renal dysfunction in patients with cirrhosis is important and may improve outcomes. Once AKI has been diagnosed, management should start immediately (**Fig. 1**). Nephrotoxic agents (eg, nonsteroidal anti-inflammatory drugs, contrast agents), vasodilators, and beta-blockers should be discontinued, and diuretic therapy should be withdrawn. Infection should be investigated and treated. AKI stage 1A (serum creatinine < 1.5 g/dL) is most often secondary to volume depletion and greater than 90% of cases resolve with risk factor management. This contrasts with only approximately 50% resolution seen in patients with AKI stage 1B.[3,37,38] Patients who present with or progress to AKI stage 1B or greater, should in addition to withdrawal of diuretics and nephrotoxic agents, and treatment of infection, receive fluid challenge of 20% to 25% intravenous albumin at 1 g/kg/d for 2 d. This step is important to rule out prerenal azotemia and is required before a diagnosis of HRS–AKI can be made. If the renal function does not improve and patients meet the additional diagnostic criteria of HRS–AKI, vasoconstrictors in combination with albumin should be initiated.

VASOCONSTRICTORS

Splanchnic vasoconstriction results in decreased portal flow, consequently portal pressure, and increased effective systemic arterial blood volume and renal blood flow. The increase in mean arterial pressure promoted by vasoconstrictors is associated with higher rates of HRS reversal.[39]

The vasoconstrictors used in the treatment of HRS-AKI include terlipressin, norepinephrine, and the combination of octreotide and midodrine (**Table 3**).

Terlipressin, a synthetic vasopressin analog, is used to treat HRS-AKI in many European and Asian countries. As a predominant vasopressin 1a agonist, terlipressin acts mainly as a splanchnic vasoconstrictor.[40] It also demonstrates mild activation of vasopressin 1b receptors, leading to the release of adrenocorticotrophic hormone and cortisol. This counteracts the relative adrenal insufficiency seen in cirrhosis.[41] Terlipressin also acts as a modest vasopressin receptor 2 agonist.

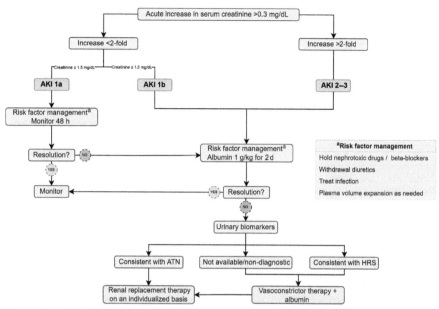

Fig. 1. Algorithm for management of acute kidney injury with cirrhosis. (*Adapted from* Simonetto DA, Gines P, Kamath PS. Hepatorenal syndrome: pathophysiology, diagnosis, and management. BMJ. 2020;370:m2687.)

Terlipressin may be administered as intravenous boluses (0.5 mg to 1 mg every 4–6 hours up to 2 mg every 4 hours) or as a continuous infusion (1 mg/d–12 mg/d). Terlipressin dose should be increased in a stepwise manner based on the response of serum creatinine for a maximum of 14 days.[38] Complete response (final serum creatinine within 0.3 mg/dL of baseline or less than 1.5 mg/dL) or partial response (improvement of AKI but final serum creatinine is $\geq$ 0.3 mg/dL of baseline) is achieved in 40% to 50% of patients. The recurrence rate of HRS–AKI is less than 20%, and in the event of recurrence, most patients respond to retreatment.[42,43]

Terlipressin is not currently Food and Drug Administration-approved in the United States, probably in part due to the rate of adverse respiratory events in patients on terlipressin.[44] The CONFIRM trial reported respiratory adverse events (including acute respiratory failure, hypoxia, pleural effusions, and pulmonary edema) in 39.5% of patients on terlipressin versus 25.3% of placebo.[45] The risk of pulmonary events may be mitigated by avoiding its use in patients with acute liver failure grade 3 or creatinine greater than or equal to 5 mg/dL, because of a lower response rate and higher risk of respiratory failure seen in these patients on sub-group analysis.[44] Further, albumin should be used with careful clinical monitoring of volume status and treatment modification or discontinuation if side effects occur. Finally, terlipressin given by continuous infusion has been associated with fewer adverse events compared with boluses administration.[46]

Norepinephrine is an intravenous systemic vasoconstrictor that works by the activation of α-1 adrenergic receptors on vascular smooth muscle cells. Norepinephrine is used as a continuous infusion (starting at 0.5 mg/h and titrated up to obtain a 10 mm Hg increase in the mean arterial blood pressure) and should be administered via a central line in an intensive care unit (ICU) setting. It has similar efficacy to terlipressin with a reversal rate of HRS–AKI ranging between 40% and 70%.[47–49]

Table 3
Vasoconstrictor therapy in the management of hepatorenal syndrome

Treatment	Route	Dose	Frequency
Terlipressin	Intravenous	1 mg; titrate if no improvement (decrease in serum creatinine by 25% by day 3) up to maximum 12 mg/d	Every 4–6 h or continuous infusion
Norepinephrine	Intravenous	0.5–3 mg/h; titrate to achieve 10 mm Hg increase in mean arterial pressure	Continuous infusion
Midodrine	Oral	5–15 mg	3 times daily
Octreotide	Subcutaneous or intravenous	100–200 μg (subcutaneous) or 50 μg/h (infusion)	3 times daily or continuous infusion

Midodrine is an oral α-1 receptor agonist. Octreotide is a somatostatin analog that inhibits glucagon (a splanchnic vasodilator) secretion and acts as a direct mesenteric vasoconstrictor. When used alone its benefit in HRS is limited.[50] However, a combination of octreotide and midodrine has a potential benefit and is the only available treatment of HRS–AKI in the United States outside the ICU.[51,52] Midodrine is dosed between 5 and 15mg three times per day and titrated based on MAP with the goal being to raise MAP by about 10 mm Hg. Octreotide may be administered either subcutaneously (100–200 mcg three times per day) or as a continuous infusion (50 mcg/h). To date, there has only been one study comparing the effect of terlipressin with midodrine and octreotide. The complete response rate in the midodrine and octreotide group was 4.8% compared with 55% with terlipressin. The overall response rate was 28.6% for midodrine and octreotide and 70.4% with terlipressin.[53] Thus, the potential benefit of midodrine and octreotide in HRS–AKI remains in question.

The role of vasoconstrictor therapy in the management of HRS–NAKI is unclear and needs to be explored in future studies.

ALBUMIN

Albumin infusion is central to the effective management of HRS–AKI and should be used in combination with vasoconstrictor therapy. Albumin acts as a volume expander and has positive cardiac ionotropic effects.[54] Studies also provide supportive evidence for its antioxidant and immunomodulatory properties.[32,55,56] Albumin may be dosed at 20 to 40 g/d based on volume and respiratory status. Excessive albumin use may result in pulmonary edema and worse outcomes, particularly when used in combination with vasoconstrictors.

TRANSJUGULAR INTRAHEPATIC PORTOSYSTEMIC SHUNT

Portal hypertension may be treated with a transjugular intrahepatic portosystemic shunt (TIPS). TIPS is beneficial in patients with cirrhosis who cannot tolerate diuretics or have diuretic-refractory ascites and as salvage, rescue, or preemptive therapy in gastroesophageal variceal hemorrhage. However, the use of TIPS in HRS–AKI remains investigational. Improvement in renal function and reduction in the activity of renin–angiotensin and sympathetic nervous system after TIPS insertion for HRS–AKI was demonstrated in one small nonrandomized study.[57] Likewise, a meta-analysis of 128 patients who underwent TIPS insertion in the setting of HRS–AKI showed improvement in serum creatinine, serum sodium, and urine output.[58] However, patients with markedly elevated bilirubin, active infection, and hepatic encephalopathy were excluded from the study. The findings may be limited to a select group of patients. TIPS is not currently recommended solely for the treatment of HRS–AKI.

RENAL REPLACEMENT THERAPY

The decision to initiate renal replacement therapy in patients with cirrhosis and AKI is based on the etiology of the AKI and the patient's transplant candidacy (**Fig. 2**). RRT has no role in the management of HRS–AKI as a stand-alone therapy.[59] However, it may be indicated in patients with treatment-refractory HRS–AKI as a bridge to liver transplantation or when the precipitating event is reversible as in selected patients with alcohol-associated hepatitis.[60,61]

LIVER TRANSPLANTATION

Liver transplantation is the definitive treatment for patients with HRS-AKI in cirrhosis. The kidney function is expected to recover after successful liver transplantation, owing to the functional nature of HRS–AKI.[62,63] However, recovery of renal function after liver transplantation is not universal and depends on multiple factors including age, comorbid conditions, and the duration of kidney injury.[64] Simultaneous liver–kidney transplantation may be indicated in these cases. In the United States, a listing policy based on consensus recommendations for a simultaneous liver–kidney transplant requires sustained AKI defined as a need for dialysis or a GFR of less than or equal to 25 mL/min for a minimum of 6 consecutive weeks.[65]

EMERGING TREATMENTS

The development of novel and effective treatment options for HRS–AKI are needed. Serelaxin is a recombinant form of the human peptide hormone relaxin-2. It increases renal perfusion by reducing renal vascular resistance and reverses endothelial dysfunction.[66] In animal models of cirrhosis, serelaxin has been shown to reduce intrahepatic vascular resistance and thus improve portal hypertension.[67] A randomized phase II study showed 65% improvement in renal perfusion from baseline in compensated cirrhotic patients treated with serelaxin.[68] Further studies are needed to elucidate the role of serelaxin in patients with HRS.

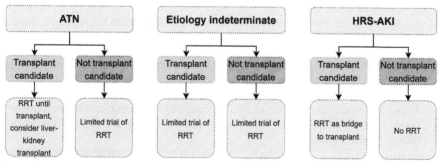

Fig. 2. Renal replacement therapy in the management of acute kidney injury in cirrhosis. Selected patients with HRS–AKI may be considered for RRT if the precipitating event is reversible, as with alcohol-associated hepatitis.

Several other drugs are currently being investigated and demonstrate promise for the treatment of HRS. These include ifetroban (a thromboxane A2/prostaglandin H2 receptor antagonist) that has successfully completed a phase II clinical trial (NCT01436500) and OCE-205 (a peptide therapeutic with a mechanism of action designed to selectively target complications of portal hypertension) that has an upcoming phase II trial (NCT05309200).

SUMMARY

Renal failure is a common and severe complication in patients with decompensated cirrhosis. HRS–AKI is a functional form of AKI in cirrhosis that confers a poor prognosis. Recently, the criteria for renal failure and HRS have been modified based on AKIN criteria with prognostic significance for cirrhosis. Our understanding of the pathophysiology of HRS–AKI has also evolved beyond circulatory dysfunction with systemic inflammation being recognized as a major factor in its development. Emphasis should remain on preventive measures for patients at risk of HRS, including appropriate use of antibiotics and albumin when indicated. Novel biomarkers such as NGAL may be useful to help determine the etiology of AKI in cirrhosis. First-line treatment of HRS–AKI is vasoconstrictor therapy and intravenous albumin. A liver transplant remains the optimal treatment and timely evaluation is critical.

CLINICS CARE POINTS

- The diagnosis of hepatorenal syndrome (HRS) is one of exclusion, and therefore should only be entertained after other possible causes of kidney injury have been ruled out.

- Classic urinary biomarkers such as urine sodium and fractional excretion of sodium, as well as the presence of renal epithelial cells and granular casts on urine microscopy, have limited accuracy in distinguishing ATN from HRS–AKI in cirrhosis. Thus, the diagnosis of ATN in patients with cirrhosis who do not respond to a fluid challenge is based on the medical history.

DISCLOSURE

The authors have no conflict of interest or funding sources to disclose.

REFERENCES

1. Garcia-Tsao G, Parikh CR, Viola A. Acute kidney injury in cirrhosis. Hepatology 2008;48(6):2064–77.
2. Fagundes C, Barreto R, Guevara M, et al. A modified acute kidney injury classification for diagnosis and risk stratification of impairment of kidney function in cirrhosis. J Hepatol 2013;59(3):474–81.
3. Piano S, Rosi S, Maresio G, et al. Evaluation of the Acute Kidney Injury Network criteria in hospitalized patients with cirrhosis and ascites. J Hepatol 2013;59(3): 482–9.
4. Arroyo V, Ginès P, Gerbes AL, et al. Definition and diagnostic criteria of refractory ascites and hepatorenal syndrome in cirrhosis. International Ascites Club. Hepatology 1996;23(1):164–76.
5. Sherman DS, Fish DN, Teitelbaum I. Assessing renal function in cirrhotic patients: Problems and pitfalls. Am J Kidney Dis 2003;41(2):269–78.
6. Bellomo R, Ronco C, Kellum JA, et al. Acute renal failure - definition, outcome measures, animal models, fluid therapy and information technology needs: the

Second International Consensus Conference of the Acute Dialysis Quality Initiative (ADQI) Group. Crit Care 2004;8(4):R204–12.

7. Mehta RL, Kellum JA, Shah SV, et al. Acute Kidney Injury Network: report of an initiative to improve outcomes in acute kidney injury. Crit Care 2007;11(2):R31.

8. Summary of recommendation Statements. Kidney Int Suppl 2012;2(1):8–12.

9. Angeli P, Gines P, Wong F, et al. Diagnosis and management of acute kidney injury in patients with cirrhosis: revised consensus recommendations of the International Club of Ascites. Gut 2015;64(4):531–7.

10. Angeli P, Garcia-Tsao G, Nadim MK, et al. News in pathophysiology, definition and classification of hepatorenal syndrome: a step beyond the International Club of Ascites (ICA) consensus document. J Hepatol 2019;71(4):811–22.

11. K/DOQI clinical practice guidelines for chronic kidney disease: evaluation, classification, and stratification. Am J Kidney Dis 2002;39(2 Suppl 1):S1–266.

12. Wong F. The evolving concept of acute kidney injury in patients with cirrhosis. Nat Rev Gastroenterol Hepatol 2015;12(12):711–9.

13. Schrier RW, Arroyo V, Bernardi M, et al. Peripheral arterial vasodilation hypothesis: a proposal for the initiation of renal sodium and water retention in cirrhosis. Hepatology 1988;8(5):1151–7.

14. Simonetto DA, Gines P, Kamath PS. Hepatorenal syndrome: pathophysiology, diagnosis, and management. BMJ 2020;370:m2687.

15. Jang JY, Kim TY, Sohn JH, et al. Relative adrenal insufficiency in chronic liver disease: its prevalence and effects on long-term mortality. Aliment Pharmacol Ther 2014;40(7):819–26.

16. Piano S, Favaretto E, Tonon M, et al. Including relative adrenal insufficiency in definition and classification of acute-on-chronic liver failure. Clin Gastroenterol Hepatol 2020;18(5):1188–96.e3.

17. Bräsen JH, Mederacke YS, Schmitz J, et al. Cholemic nephropathy causes acute kidney injury and is Accompanied by loss of Aquaporin 2 in Collecting Ducts. Hepatology 2019;69(5):2107–19.

18. Umgelter A, Reindl W, Wagner KS, et al. Effects of plasma expansion with albumin and paracentesis on haemodynamics and kidney function in critically ill cirrhotic patients with tense ascites and hepatorenal syndrome: a prospective uncontrolled trial. Crit Care 2008;12(1):R4.

19. Martín-Llahí M, Guevara M, Torre A, et al. Prognostic importance of the cause of renal failure in patients with cirrhosis. Gastroenterology 2011;140(2):488–96.e4.

20. Verna EC, Brown RS, Farrand E, et al. Urinary neutrophil gelatinase-associated lipocalin predicts mortality and identifies acute kidney injury in cirrhosis. Dig Dis Sci 2012;57(9):2362–70.

21. Huelin P, Solà E, Elia C, et al. Neutrophil gelatinase-associated lipocalin for assessment of acute kidney injury in cirrhosis: a prospective study. Hepatology 2019;70(1):319–33.

22. Fagundes C, Pépin MN, Guevara M, et al. Urinary neutrophil gelatinase-associated lipocalin as biomarker in the differential diagnosis of impairment of kidney function in cirrhosis. J Hepatol 2012;57(2):267–73.

23. Decavele AS, Dhondt L, De Buyzere ML, et al. Increased urinary neutrophil gelatinase associated lipocalin in urinary tract infections and leukocyturia. Clin Chem Lab Med 2011;49(6):999–1003.

24. Liu Y, Guo W, Zhang J, et al. Urinary interleukin 18 for Detection of acute kidney injury: a meta-analysis. Am J Kidney Dis 2013;62(6):1058–67.

25. Ariza X, Solà E, Elia C, et al. Analysis of a urinary biomarker panel for clinical outcomes assessment in cirrhosis. PLoS One 2015;10(6):e0128145.

26. Puthumana J, Ariza X, Belcher JM, et al. Urine interleukin 18 and lipocalin 2 are biomarkers of acute tubular necrosis in patients with cirrhosis: a systematic review and meta-analysis. Clin Gastroenterol Hepatol 2017;15(7):1003–13.e3.

27. Ginès A, Escorsell A, Ginès P, et al. Incidence, predictive factors, and prognosis of the hepatorenal syndrome in cirrhosis with ascites. Gastroenterology 1993; 105(1):229–36.

28. Wong F, Jepsen P, Watson H, et al. Un-precipitated acute kidney injury is uncommon among stable patients with cirrhosis and ascites. Liver Int 2018;38(10): 1785–92.

29. Ginès P, Titó L, Arroyo V, et al. Randomized comparative study of therapeutic paracentesis with and without intravenous albumin in cirrhosis. Gastroenterology 1988;94(6):1493–502.

30. Bernardi M, Caraceni P, Navickis RJ, et al. Albumin infusion in patients undergoing large-volume paracentesis: a meta-analysis of randomized trials. Hepatology 2012;55(4):1172–81.

31. Fernández J, Monteagudo J, Bargallo X, et al. A randomized unblinded pilot study comparing albumin versus hydroxyethyl starch in spontaneous bacterial peritonitis. Hepatology 2005;42(3):627–34.

32. Zhang W-J, Frei B. Albumin selectively inhibits TNFα-induced expression of vascular cell adhesion molecule-1 in human aortic endothelial cells. Cardiovasc Res 2002;55(4):820–9.

33. Chen T-A, Tsao Y-C, Chen A, et al. Effect of intravenous albumin on endotoxin removal, cytokines, and nitric oxide production in patients with cirrhosis and spontaneous bacterial peritonitis. Scand J Gastroenterol 2009;44(5):619–25.

34. Follo A, Llovet JM, Navasa M, et al. Renal impairment after spontaneous bacterial peritonitis in cirrhosis: incidence, clinical course, predictive factors and prognosis. Hepatology 1994;20(6):1495–501.

35. Fernández J, Navasa M, Planas R, et al. Primary prophylaxis of spontaneous bacterial peritonitis Delays hepatorenal syndrome and improves survival in cirrhosis. Gastroenterology 2007;133(3):818–24.

36. Kamal F, Khan MA, Khan Z, et al. Rifaximin for the prevention of spontaneous bacterial peritonitis and hepatorenal syndrome in cirrhosis: a systematic review and meta-analysis. Eur J Gastroenterol Hepatol 2017;29(10):1109–17.

37. Huelin P, Piano S, Solà E, et al. Validation of a staging system for acute kidney injury in patients with cirrhosis and association with acute-on-chronic liver failure. Clin Gastroenterol Hepatol 2017;15(3):438–45.e5.

38. EASL Clinical Practice Guidelines for the management of patients with decompensated cirrhosis. J Hepatol 2018;69(2):406–60.

39. Velez JC, Nietert PJ. Therapeutic response to vasoconstrictors in hepatorenal syndrome parallels increase in mean arterial pressure: a pooled analysis of clinical trials. Am J Kidney Dis 2011;58(6):928–38.

40. Jamil K, Pappas SC, Devarakonda KR. In vitro binding and receptor-mediated activity of terlipressin at vasopressin receptors V(1) and V(2). J Exp Pharmacol 2017;10:1–7.

41. Tanoue A, Ito S, Honda K, et al. The vasopressin V1b receptor critically regulates hypothalamic-pituitary-adrenal axis activity under both stress and resting conditions. J Clin Invest 2004;113(2):302–9.

42. Boyer TD, Medicis JJ, Pappas SC, et al. A randomized, placebo-controlled, double-blind study to confirm the reversal of hepatorenal syndrome type 1 with terlipressin: the REVERSE trial design. Open Access J Clin Trials 2012;4:39–49.

43. Martín-Llahí M, Pépin MN, Guevara M, et al. Terlipressin and albumin vs albumin in patients with cirrhosis and hepatorenal syndrome: a randomized study. Gastroenterology 2008;134(5):1352–9.

44. Belcher JM, Parada XV, Simonetto DA, et al. Terlipressin and the treatment of hepatorenal syndrome: How the CONFIRM trial Moves the story Forward. Am J Kidney Dis 2022;79(5):737–45.

45. Wong F, Pappas SC, Curry MP, et al. Terlipressin plus albumin for the treatment of type 1 hepatorenal syndrome. New Engl J Med 2021;384(9):818–28.

46. Cavallin M, Piano S, Romano A, et al. Terlipressin given by continuous intravenous infusion versus intravenous boluses in the treatment of hepatorenal syndrome: a randomized controlled study. Hepatology 2016;63(3):983–92.

47. Alessandria C, Ottobrelli A, Debernardi-Venon W, et al. Noradrenalin vs terlipressin in patients with hepatorenal syndrome: a prospective, randomized, unblinded, pilot study. J Hepatol 2007;47(4):499–505.

48. Sharma P, Kumar A, Shrama BC, et al. An open label, pilot, randomized controlled trial of noradrenaline versus terlipressin in the treatment of type 1 hepatorenal syndrome and predictors of response. Am J Gastroenterol 2008;103(7): 1689–97.

49. Singh V, Ghosh S, Singh B, et al. Noradrenaline vs. terlipressin in the treatment of hepatorenal syndrome: a randomized study. J Hepatol 2012;56(6):1293–8.

50. Angeli P, Volpin R, Piovan D, et al. Acute effects of the oral administration of midodrine, an α-adrenergic agonist, on renal hemodynamics and renal function in cirrhotic patients with ascites. Hepatology 1998;28(4):937–43.

51. Angeli P, Volpin R, Gerunda G, et al. Reversal of type 1 hepatorenal syndrome with the administration of midodrine and octreotide. Hepatology 1999;29(6): 1690–7.

52. Wong F, Pantea L, Sniderman K. Midodrine, octreotide, albumin, and TIPS in selected patients with cirrhosis and type 1 hepatorenal syndrome. Hepatology 2004;40(1):55–64.

53. Cavallin M, Kamath PS, Merli M, et al. Terlipressin plus albumin versus midodrine and octreotide plus albumin in the treatment of hepatorenal syndrome: a randomized trial. Hepatology 2015;62(2):567–74.

54. Bortoluzzi A, Ceolotto G, Gola E, et al. Positive cardiac inotropic effect of albumin infusion in rodents with cirrhosis and ascites: molecular mechanisms. Hepatology 2013;57(1):266–76.

55. Stocker R, Glazer AN, Ames BN. Antioxidant activity of albumin-bound bilirubin. Proc Natl Acad Sci 1987;84(16):5918–22.

56. Cantin AM, Paquette B, Richter M, et al. Albumin-mediated regulation of cellular glutathione and nuclear factor kappa B activation. Am J Respir Crit Care Med 2000;162(4 Pt 1):1539–46.

57. Guevara M, Ginès P, Bandi JC, et al. Transjugular intrahepatic portosystemic shunt in hepatorenal syndrome: effects on renal function and vasoactive systems. Hepatology 1998;28(2):416–22.

58. Song T, Rössle M, He F, et al. Transjugular intrahepatic portosystemic shunt for hepatorenal syndrome: a systematic review and meta-analysis. Dig Liver Dis 2018;50(4):323–30.

59. Zhang Z, Maddukuri G, Jaipaul N, et al. Role of renal replacement therapy in patients with type 1 hepatorenal syndrome receiving combination treatment of vasoconstrictor plus albumin. J Crit Care 2015;30(5):969–74.

60. Lenhart A, Hussain S, Salgia R. Chances of renal recovery or liver transplantation after Hospitalization for alcoholic liver disease requiring dialysis. Dig Dis Sci 2018;63(10):2800–9.
61. Jones BE, Allegretti AS, Pose E, et al. Renal replacement therapy for acute kidney injury in severe alcohol-associated hepatitis as a bridge to transplant or recovery. Dig Dis Sci 2022;67(2):697–707.
62. EASL clinical practice guidelines on the management of ascites, spontaneous bacterial peritonitis, and hepatorenal syndrome in cirrhosis. J Hepatol 2010; 53(3):397–417.
63. Runyon BA. Management of adult patients with ascites due to cirrhosis: an update. Hepatology 2009;49(6):2087–107.
64. Israni AK, Xiong H, Liu J, et al. Predicting end-stage renal disease after liver transplant. Am J Transpl 2013;13(7):1782–92.
65. Organ Procurement and Transplantation Network. Policies. 2022. Available at: https://optn.transplant.hrsa.gov/media/eavh5bf3/optn_policies.pdf
66. Conrad KP. Unveiling the vasodilatory actions and mechanisms of relaxin. Hypertension 2010;56(1):2–9.
67. Snowdon VK, Lachlan NJ, Hoy AM, et al. Serelaxin as a potential treatment for renal dysfunction in cirrhosis: Preclinical evaluation and results of a randomized phase 2 trial. Plos Med 2017;14(2):e1002248.
68. Stine JG, Wang J, Cornella SL, et al. Treatment of type-1 hepatorenal syndrome with Pentoxifylline: a randomized placebo controlled clinical trial. Ann Hepatol 2018;17(2):300–6.

Portopulmonary Hypertension

Yu Kuang Lai, MD[a], Paul Y. Kwo, MD[b],*

KEYWORDS

- Portopulmonary hypertension • Pulmonary hypertension • Liver transplant

KEY POINTS

- Pulmonary hypertension (PH) was historically defined by an elevated mean pulmonary artery pressure (mPAP) $\geq$25 mm Hg on right heart catheterization though recent classification data have now defined the threshold for PH as having an mPAP of > 20 mm Hg at rest
- The goal of therapy is to improve symptoms and/or optimize pulmonary hemodynamics such that the patient can undergo a liver transplant safely.
- Patients are eligible for portopulmonary hypertension (PoPH) model for end-stage liver disease (MELD) exception points provided that their initial right heart catheterization (RHC) is consistent with the hemodynamic definition of PoPH with a mean pulmonary artery pressure (mPAP) > 35 mm Hg, and were able to attain mPAP <35 mm Hg and pulmonary vascular resistance (PVR) of <400 dyn-s-cm^{-5} or 5 WU on pulmonary arterial hypertension (PAH) targeted therapy or mPAP between 35 mm Hg and 45 mm Hg on PAH targeted therapy as long as the PVR is normalized (<3 WU or 240 dyn-s-cm^{-5}) and right ventricle function is adequate.
- Although liver transplantation provides benefits for those with PoPH, the question remains whether all those with PoPH should be offered MELD exception points over those with decompensated liver disease or should a more selective approach be considered.

INTRODUCTION

Portopulmonary hypertension (PoPH) is a well-recognized complication of portal hypertension with or without cirrhosis and is classified as a subset of pulmonary arterial hypertension (PAH). Identification of PoPH is crucial as it has a major impact on prognosis and liver transplant candidacy. Survival of PoPH patients is worse than in other forms of pulmonary hypertension (PH) despite having a better hemodynamic profile, possibly attributed to underlying liver disease. Symptoms can range from asymptomatic to features of right heart failure that often can be indistinguishable from decompensated liver disease. Early diagnosis of PoPH relies on a high index of suspicion with thorough history taking and evaluation. Echocardiogram is the initial screening tool of choice and the

[a] Pulmonary, Allergy and Critical Care, Department of Medicine, Stanford University, 300 Pasteur Drive, Room H3143, Palo Alto, CA 94304, USA; [b] Stanford University School of Medicine, 430 Broadway, Pavilion C, 3rd Floor, Redwood City, CA 94063, USA
* Corresponding author.
E-mail address: pkwo@stanford.edu

Clin Liver Dis 27 (2023) 71–84
https://doi.org/10.1016/j.cld.2022.08.002
1089-3261/23/© 2022 Elsevier Inc. All rights reserved.

liver.theclinics.com

1 PAH
    1.1 Idiopathic PAH
    1.2 Heritable PAH
    1.3 Drug- and toxin-induced PAH
    1.4 PAH associated with:
        1.4.1 Connective tissue disease
        1.4.2 HIV infection
        1.4.3 Portal hypertension
        1.4.4 Congenital heart disease
        1.4.5 Schistosomiasis
    1.5 PAH long-term responders to calcium channel blockers
    1.6 PAH with overt features of venous/capillaries (PVOD/PCH) involvement
    1.7 Persistent PH of the newborn syndrome
2 PH due to left heart disease
    2.1 PH due to heart failure with preserved LVEF
    2.2 PH due to heart failure with reduced LVEF
    2.3 Valvular heart disease
    2.4 Congenital/acquired cardiovascular conditions leading to post-capillary PH
3 PH due to lung diseases and/or hypoxia
    3.1 Obstructive lung disease
    3.2 Restrictive lung disease
    3.3 Other lung disease with mixed restrictive/obstructive pattern
    3.4 Hypoxia without lung disease
    3.5 Developmental lung disorders
4 PH due to pulmonary artery obstructions
    4.1 Chronic thromboembolic PH
    4.2 Other pulmonary artery obstructions
5 PH with unclear and/or multifactorial mechanisms
    5.1 Hematological disorders
    5.2 Systemic and metabolic disorders
    5.3 Others
    5.4 Complex congenital heart disease

Fig. 1. World Health Organization clinical classification of pulmonary hypertension. LVEF, left ventricular ejection fraction; PAH, pulmonary arterial hypertension; PCH, pulmonary capillary hemangiomatosis; PH, pulmonary hypertension; PVOD, pulmonary veno-occlusive disease.

patient should proceed to right heart catheterization (RHC) for confirmation. PAH-directed therapy is the treatment of choice, allowing the patient to achieve a hemodynamic threshold to undergo liver transplant safely. Liver transplantation (LT) can address the portal hypertension but it should not be considered as a treatment for PoPH in those who otherwise do not meet liver transplant criteria. This article covers the epidemiology of PoPH, factors associated with morbidity and mortality, and its pathophysiology. We outline the diagnostic workup, with an emphasis on echocardiogram findings and an in-depth interpretation of hemodynamic data. Finally, we review the current practice guidance evidence in caring for those with PoPH and therapeutic options.

DEFINITION

PH was historically defined by an elevated mean pulmonary artery pressure (mPAP) $\geq$25 mm Hg on RHC though recent classification data have now defined the threshold for PH as having an mPAP of > 20 mm Hg at rest.[1] PH is classified into five clinical subgroups based on histologic similarities, hemodynamic definition, and therapeutic management (**Fig. 1, Table 1**). PoPH is a subset of World Health Organization

Table 1 Hemodynamic definitions of pulmonary hypertension		
Definition	**RHC Findings**	**WHO PH Groups**
Pre-capillary PH	mPAP >20 mm Hg PAWP <15 mm Hg PVR >3 WU	1,3,4 and 5
Post-capillary PH	mPAP >20 mm Hg PAWP >15 mm Hg PVR <3 WU	2 and 5
Combined pre- and post Capillary PH	mPAP >20 mm Hg PAWP >15 mm Hg PVR >3 WU	2 and 5

Abbreviations: mPAP, mean pulmonary arterial pressure; PAWP, pulmonary arterial wedge pressure; PVR, pulmonary vascular resistance; RHC, right heart catheterization; WU, wood Units.

(WHO) group 1 PH, defined as precapillary PH or PAH, hemodynamically characterized by a map of greater than 20 mm Hg, pulmonary vascular resistance (PVR) of greater 3 WU or 240 dyn-s-cm^{-5} and a pulmonary arterial wedge pressure (PAWP) of less than 15 mm Hg, associated with cirrhotic or non-cirrhotic portal hypertension.

Epidemiology

The prevalence of PoPH has not been precisely defined and reports vary depending on the population studied and hemodynamic definition. Importantly, some studies have noted high pulmonary artery pressures but without documented elevated PVR of greater than 3 WU or 240 dyn-s-cm^{-5}, which is prerequisite hemodynamic criteria to fulfill the definition of PoPH. For example, data analysis from the Organ Procurement and Transplant Network for PoPH model for end-stage liver disease (MELD) exception during the period 2006 to 2012 showed that among patient awarded with exception points, only 47.1% of patients actually met hemodynamic criteria for PoPH.[2] Most reports are derived from patients presenting with end-stage liver disease with screening for PoPH as a part of a transplant evaluation. Multiple series have estimated a prevalence of PoPH in those with cirrhosis ranging from 2% in chronic liver disease patients to 16% in those with cirrhosis and listed for LT. In a classic autopsy study of 17,901 patients, the prevalence of histopathological findings suggestive of PoPH was reported at 0.73% of patients with cirrhosis compared with a prevalence of 0.13% in those without cirrhosis.[3] One large trial reported a prevalence of 5% as documented by RHC in a screening program for those with primary biliary cirrhosis.[4] Similarly, a wide range of prevalence rates of PoPH has been reported in those with pulmonary artery hypertension with 1 large PH registry (REVEAL registry) estimating the prevalence of PoPH at 5.4% of PAH cases.[5]

With regard to risk factors, one case-control study has suggested female gender and autoimmune liver disease are associated with an increased risk of PoPH and primary biliary cholangitis has also been associated with increased risk.[6,7] These findings are consistent with what is observed in patients with idiopathic pulmonary artery hypertension where female gender is also a risk factor. Finally, the severity of cirrhosis as assessed by Child Pugh Score or MELD score does not seem to correlate with the presence or severity of PoPH.

Natural History

The survival of those with PoPH is poor. A recent registry from the United Kingdom in 110 individuals from 2001 to 2010 with PoPH hypertension noted survival rates at 1, 3, and 5 years of 85%, 60%, and 35% in a population largely comprised of those with alcohol-associated liver disease and viral hepatitis. Severity of cirrhosis or the presence of cirrhosis, pulmonary hemodynamics, or year of diagnosis was not associated with survival.[8] Another large study examined 174 individuals with PoPH from 2006 to 2009 and noted reduced survival in those with PoPH compared with idiopathic PH or other forms of PH with a 5-year survival rate of 40% versus 64%.[9]

Pathogenesis

The pathogenesis of PoPH has yet to be established but there are likely multiple etiologic factors involved. The most widely accepted theory postulates that in the presence of portal hypertension there is the formation of portosystemic shunting, facilitating the bypass of liver metabolism of various vasoactive metabolites such as endothelin-1, serotonin, and glucagon, leading to direct or indirect pulmonary endothelium and arterial smooth muscle injury.[10,11] A localized inflammatory response or thromboembolic phenomenon has also been postulated but there has been scant evidence to support these hypotheses. Chronic exposure to a high flow state could cause shear stress on the endothelial cell, provoking remodeling of the pulmonary vascular bed, featuring a proliferation of smooth muscle cells and marked intima and medial thickening, but whether this phenomenon is also responsible for the hyperdynamic state intrinsic to underlying liver disease is less clear.[12,13] Ultimately, these pathologic changes results in progressive obliteration of small pulmonary arteries, subsequently causes an elevation of PVR that is poorly tolerated by the right ventricle (RV), leading to right ventricular failure.

Evaluation

A detailed history and physical examination are important in screening for PoPH. As the clinical manifestation of PoPH is indistinguishable from other forms of PH, history taking should also include assessing other risk factors for PH such as prior methamphetamine use, history of connective tissue disease, left heart disease, interstitial lung disease, sleep apnea, and pulmonary embolism.

Symptoms of PoPH range from asymptomatic to features of right ventricular failure, commonly present with dyspnea or chest pain on exertion, dizziness, syncope, palpitation and generalized swelling. Notably, these symptoms are shared with decompensated liver disease and associated clinical manifestations such as hepatopulmonary syndrome and hepatic hydrothorax and are therefore rather nonspecific. Anasarca, ascites, pulsatile hepatomegaly, elevated jugular venous pressure, loud pulmonic S2, and holosystolic murmur from tricuspid regurgitation, accentuated by inspiration can be appreciated on physical examination.

The electrocardiogram (ECG) may show presence of right atrial or RV enlargement, right axis shift, or evidence of RV strain pattern. However, a normal ECG does not exclude PH. Enlarged cardiac silhouette on chest imaging and pulmonary artery on computed tomography (CT) should prompt further workup for PH.

Screening and Diagnostic Strategy

RHC is the gold standard diagnostic tool for PH. However, it is usually not the initial diagnostic step of choice, barring from its invasiveness and availability. Consequently, transthoracic echocardiogram (TTE) remains the most cost-effective and practical

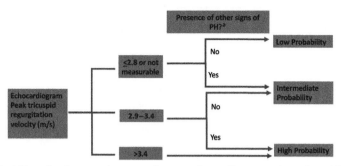

Fig. 2. Probability of pulmonary hypertension on echocardiogram using tricuspid regurgitation velocity.[a]See Signs from at least two different categories (Ventricle, Pulmonary artery, Inferiorvena cava/Right atrium) should be present to alter the level of probability for PH. PH, pulmonary hypertension.

screening tool for PH. As the symptoms of PoPH may be subtle and nonspecific, TTE should not only be considered in the patient with symptoms but is also a mandatory workup for patients undergoing liver transplant evaluation, regardless of symptoms.

Traditionally, right ventricular systolic pressure (RVSP) is the common surrogate on TTE to determine if the patient warrants an RHC for confirmation. The RVSP is estimated by using the simplified Bernoulli equation, derived from peak tricuspid regurgitant velocity (TRV) and estimated right atrial pressure. There are several factors that could affect the measurement of RVSP. The accuracy of RVSP weighs heavily on operator experience, proper visualization, and adequate Doppler alignment on TR jet. Hepatomegaly or large ascites may jeopardize proper imaging acquisition hence affect the accuracy of RVSP estimation.[14] TRV can be accentuated by hyperdynamic state from the liver disease which can overestimate RVSP. These limitations explain the discrepancy observed between the RVSP and the actual pulmonary arterial systolic pressure (PASP) measured by RHC, and the resulting the correlation between RVSP and mean pulmonary arterial pressure (mPAP) is modest at best.[3,15–18] As such, a precise cutoff value of RVSP for which RHC should be considered does not exist and the threshold to perform RHC varies among institutions and society guidelines.[19] For example, the American Association for Study of Liver Disease recommend to proceed with RHC if RVSP is ≥ 45 mm Hg,[20] whereas The International Liver Transplant Society guidelines recommend an RHC in a patient with RVSP >50 mm Hg and/or evidence of right ventricular hypertrophy or dysfunction.[21] Given the limitation of RVSP, the sixth World Symposium on PH has recommended to assess the probability of PH by using the combination of TRV and presence of other signs of PH on TTE, rather than relying on estimated RVSP alone.[22] Patients with moderate-to-high probability of PH on TTE should proceed to RHC for confirmation (**Fig. 2, Table 2**).

Diagnosis

As with other forms of PH, RHC is mandatory in making the diagnosis PoPH. As discussed previously, PoPH is a subset of WHO group 1 PH, a vasculopathy exquisitely involved in the precapillary region, hemodynamically characterized by an elevated mPAP of >20 mm Hg, PVR > 3 WU or 240 dyn-s-cm^{-5} and normal PAWP of <15 mm Hg. The relationships between these variables are illustrated by the equation below:

$$mPAP = cardiac\ output\ (CO) \times PVR + PAWP.$$

Table 2
Signs of pulmonary hypertension on echocardiogram in addition to tricuspid regurgitation velocity measurement

Ventricles	RV/LV basal diameter>1	Flattening of the interventricular septum	
Pulmonary Artery	PA diameter > 25 mm	Early diastolic pulmonary regurgitation velocity > 2.2 m/s	RV outflow Doppler acceleration < 105 ms and/or mid systolic notching
Inferior vena cava and right atrium	RA end -systolic area > 18 cm^2	IVC diameter > 21 mm with the decreased inspiratory collapse	

Abbreviations: IVC, inferior vena cava; LV, left ventricle; PA, pulmonary artery; RA, right ventricle.

From the above equation, one can appreciate that, apart from elevated PVR, high CO and PAWP can also elevate mPAP. Conditions that have a known association with liver diseases such as high CO and volume overload can also cause an elevated mPAP despite PVR being normal (**Table 3**). In other words, an isolated increase in mPAP is insufficient to diagnose PoPH. Careful evaluation of RHC metrics is crucial to distinguish PoPH from other causes of PH, as the management and prognosis of these entities are very different.[17,23] In practice, it is not uncommon to find these conditions concomitantly in those with advanced liver disease, thus making the hemodynamic interpretation and diagnosis of PoPH more challenging. To avoid these confounders, if possible, RHC should be performed once the confounding factors, such as volume overload or sepsis, are optimized. Lastly, as PoPH is hemodynamically indistinguishable from other WHO group 1 PH (see **Fig. 1**, **Table 1**), a thorough evaluation and appropriate investigation (eg, drug toxin screen, connective tissue disease serology) should be conducted to exclude alternative causes of WHO group 1 PH.

Management

General
The goal of therapy is to improve symptoms and/or optimize pulmonary hemodynamics such that the patient can undergo the liver transplant safely. As with other forms of PH, volume status optimization is paramount to support the decompensated RV. Sodium restriction and diuretics therapy are standard interventions but should be cautiously implemented in a patient with advanced liver disease to avoid acute kidney injury, and electrolyte abnormalities though achieving euvolemic status in these patients can be challenging.[24] Hypoxemia, hypercarbia, and acidosis are known insults with worsening PVR and should be addressed appropriately. Use of beta-blockers may be beneficial for patients with portal hypertension, but its use in the setting of moderate to severe PoPH and/or decompensated RV function is generally discouraged due to its negative chronotropic effect.[25,26]

Pulmonary vasodilators
There are 13 US Food and Drug Administration (FDA)-approved PAH-targeted therapies available and are categorized based on their mechanism of action, namely nitric oxide, endothelin, and prostacyclin pathway (**Table 4**). The principle mechanism is to reduce PVR, restore flow through vasodilation, inhibit vascular remodeling, and ultimately improve RV function. Unfortunately, PoPH is routinely excluded from major

Table 3
Right heart catheterization profile for patient with elevated mean pulmonary arterial pressures

Clinical Condition	Mean Pulmonary Arterial Pressure	Cardiac Output	Pulmonary Vascular Resistance	Pulmonary Arterial Wedge Pressure
Portopulmonary Hypertension	↑	↓/N	↑	↓
Volume Overload	↑	↑/N	N	↑
Hyperdynamic State[a]	↑	↑	↓	↓/N

Down arrow, decreased; N, normal; Up arrow, increased.
[a] Sepsis, anemia, cirrhosis, hyperthyroidism.

PH clinical trials,[27] hence the use of PAH-targeted therapy in PoPH are limited to retrospective analysis, case series, and provider experience. Nonetheless, these agents are efficacious in improving hemodynamics, allowing a bridge to LT.

Nitric oxide pathway

Nitric oxide is a potent mediator in maintaining pulmonary vasoregulation and is produced predominantly in vascular endothelium.[28] Phosphodiesterase-5 inhibitors and riociguat promote vasodilation by increasing the bioavailability and sensitivity of nitric oxide through a different molecular target and ultimately inhibit smooth muscle cell contraction. Their use in PoPH is generally safe[29–31] and well tolerated. However, these agents are also potent systemic vasodilators and their use may be severely limited or prohibitive in PoPH patients with low blood pressure.

Endothelin pathway

Endothelin is known for its potent vasoconstriction property on the vasculature and promotes a remodeling process by mediation through endothelin A receptor.[32] Endothelin receptor antagonist (ERA) agents have shown to improve functional class and time to clinical worsening. The primary safety concern with ERA agents that have been reported is hepatotoxicity hence regular monitoring of liver tests is advised. The transaminitis associated with ERAs is usually transient and reversible with dose adjustment or discontinuation and is more often described in bosentan than in macitentan or ambrisentan.[33,34] That being said, one should be cautious in the use of such agents in Child-Pugh C class cirrhosis patients as these patients are excluded in the study involved with ERA due to concern of high risk for drug-induced liver injury.

Macitentan for the treatment of portopulmonary hypertension (PORTICO) was the first randomized controlled trial performed exclusively in PoPH using macitentan and has shown a 35% reduction in PVR and improvement in the cardiac index after 12 weeks of therapy. Though there was no improvement in functional class or walk distance observed, there were no significant hepatic safety concerns. One confounder is that most of the patients in the trial were on other-background PAH therapies.[35]

Prostacyclin pathway

Prostacyclin was the first FDA-approved PAH therapy in 1995 and has since revolutionized the outlook of PAH,[36] a disease previously perceived with ominous outcomes. It acts as a potent vasodilator on the smooth muscle cell. In addition, it attenuates vascular remodeling through its anti-inflammatory, antiproliferative, and antiplatelet properties. It can be delivered via 4 routes: oral, inhaled, subcutaneous, or intravenous.[37] Intravenous epoprostenol is considered the most potent therapeutic agent

Table 4			
Current FDA-approved targeted PAH therapy and mode of administration			
Pathway	Drug Class	Mode of Administration	Drug Name
Nitric Oxide	Phosphodiesterase type 5 inhibitor	Oral	Sildenafil
			Tadalafil
	Soluble guanylate cyclase stimulator	Oral	Riociguat
Endothelin	Endothelin receptor antagonists	Oral	Ambrisentan
			Bosentan
			Macitentan
Prostacyclin	Prostacyclin analog	Inhaled	Treprostinil
			Iloprost
		Intravenous	Epoprostenol
			Treprostinil
		Oral	Treprostinil
		Subcutaneous	Treprostinil
	Prostacyclin IP Receptor Agonist	Oral	Selexipag

for PAH and offers stabilization of the disease in a short time frame. However, these attributes should balance against its significant side effect profile such as thrombocytopenia, splenomegaly, and risks of catheter-related adverse events including bloodstream infection and thrombosis. Furthermore, psychosocial contraindications should be carefully screened for as the accurate drug administration and safety rely heavily on patient's understanding of the delivery device and family support. Therefore, parenteral therapy is strictly reserved for highly selected individuals with high-risk features such as syncope, severe RV dysfunction, and patient with rapid progression of the disease.

Special consideration in using pulmonary arterial hypertension targeted therapy in portopulmonary hypertension

The treatment strategy for PoPH has been adopted from treatment algorithms for other forms of PAH, with specific considerations. For example, it is standard of care to introduce upfront combination PAH therapy upon diagnosis, but the safety of such an approach for PoPH has not been established and may not be feasible in decompensated liver disease, as vasodilators are known to decrease systemic resistance that may potentially exacerbate the preexisting hyperdynamic circulatory state. ERAs are known to cause fluid retention which may limit its use as the first agent of choice for a patient with challenging volume status. Oral and inhaled PAH target therapy generally takes weeks to months to achieve a clinically meaningful effect. These agents thus may not be ideal for a patient with sensitive transplant windows, who needs expedited PoPH optimization to proceed to LT. Given these nuances, clinicians should be aware of these challenges, understanding the selection of agent, route of administration, and escalation strategy requires extensive collaboration among specialists and close follow-up, and thus is best managed by the PH center of expertise.

Liver Transplant

PoPH was once considered as a contraindication for liver transplant given its high perioperative mortality.[23] With the advent of PAH targeted therapy, liver transplant is now permissible as long as patients are able to meet the certain hemodynamic threshold. The landmark paper by Krowka and colleagues[23] outlined the framework for the hemodynamic threshold to allow safe transplants and is widely accepted in current practice.[20,21]

Traditionally, the severity and perioperative mortality of PoPH is stratified by mPAP. This is based on a retrospective study in 2000 by Krowka and colleagues[23] where PoPH with mPAP of >50 mm Hg, 35 < mPAP <50 mm Hg, and <35 mm Hg was associated with 100%, 50%, 0% cardiopulmonary mortality, respectively. Since then, the treatment goal has been focusing on reducing mPAP to < 35 mm Hg to meet transplant eligibility. Acknowledging that the severity of PoPH can progress and laboratory MELD score does not accurately reflect overall mortality risk in a patient with PoPH, PoPH MELD exception criteria were established in 2006 with the intent to prioritize liver transplant in these patients before their cardiopulmonary risk become prohibitive to undergo a safe liver transplant. Patients are eligible for PoPH MELD exception points provided that their initial RHC is consistent with the hemodynamic definition of PoPH with an mPAP > 35 mm Hg, and were able to attain mPAP <35 mm Hg and PVR of <400 dyn-s-cm^{-5} or 5 WU after 12 weeks of PAH targeted therapy.

However, a growing body of evidence has shown that PVR is a more reliable marker in predicting overall mortality, perioperative risk, and graft failure than mPAP.[38–40] Numerous studies have shown that a safe liver transplant is feasible and has similar LT outcomes even if mPAP is > 35 mm Hg with a normal PVR (<240 dyn-s-cm^{-5} or <3 WU) and an adequate RV function,[17,41] as patients with these hemodynamic profiles are likely to have volume overload and/or hyperdynamic circulatory status as the cause of elevated mPAP, rather than originated from pulmonary arterial vasculopathy, or PoPH, per se.[17,39,42,43] Moreover, although PoPH is expected to improve with PAH targeted therapy, mPAP may remain persistently elevated despite normalized PVR due to concomitant increase in CO and/or PAWP, such patients may also undergo transplant safely as well.[17,41] In response to these findings, PoPH MELD exception criteria was revised and modified in October 2021https://optn.transplant.hrsa.gov/media/3927/further_enhancements_nlrb_pc.pdf, where patient previously excluded from exception pathway due to their mPAP remained between 35 mm Hg and 45 mm Hg despite on PAH targeted therapy, are now qualified to receive exception points, as long as the PVR is normalized (<3 WU or 240 dyn-s-cm^{-5}) and RV function is adequate.[44] This again underscores the importance of obtaining a high-quality RHC to allow a comprehensive assessment of pre-LT hemodynamic evaluation, is the best way to provide appropriate treatment strategy and transplant risk stratification. **Fig. 3** summarized the algorithm in the management of PoPH, incorporating hemodynamic studies.

Clinical course of PoPH immediately after LT remains unpredictable. Although some studies have shown improvement of PoPH, allowing discontinuation of PAH targeted therapy after LT,[41,45] others have reported progressive RV failure needing additional PAH targeted therapy, or rapid cardiopulmonary collapse during LT, despite PoPH being well treated at the time of LT.[46,47] Retrospective studies have observed these adverse outcome tends to occur within 6 months after LT.[42,48,49] Therefore, discontinuation or tapering PAH targeted therapy within this time frame is strongly discouraged, and close follow-up is highly recommended.

Whereas hepatopulmonary syndrome has a clear indication for LT, with survival benefits, whether this life-saving intervention applies to PoPH remains more contentious. A study by Saad and colleagues comparing the survival rate between PoPH patients who underwent LT versus patients treated by PAH therapy alone showed a significant 1,3,5-year survival difference: 95%,8% vs 74.5%, 90.9% vs 59.3%, 90.9% vs 35.9%, respectively. Savale and colleagues also reported promising survival benefits for PoPH patients who underwent LT as compared with the group who were not transplanted,

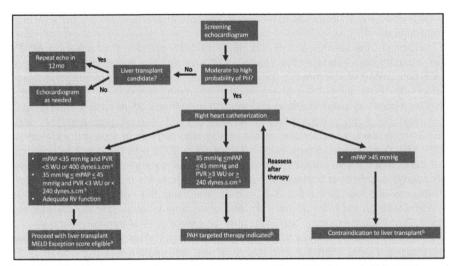

Fig. 3. PoPH screening evaluation and treatment algorithm. [a]Eligible only if PoPH showed mPAP greater than 35 mm Hg upon initial (pre-treatment) right heart catheterization. [b]Referral to PH center for therapy is highly recommended. mPAP, mean pulmonary arterial pressure; PVR, pulmonary vascular resistance.

irrespective of MELD score or Child-Pugh stage.[50] The survival benefit observed from these studies raise the question of whether LT should be offered to PoPH patient even without indication for transplant per current guideline. In contrast, Ceba and colleagues described modest posttransplant survival rates for PoPH in 1-, 3-, and 5-year at 72%, 63%, and 60% respectively.[51] These conflicting observations are likely driven by considerable heterogeneity among the studied population, the difference in comorbidities, and the severity of the liver disease. These disparate findings are also reflected on clinical practice. A survey conducted by Dubrock and colleagues in 35 transplant centers illustrates the variability in practice patterns and perception among hepatologists and PH physicians.[19] Hepatologists are more likely than PH physicians, to agreed that PoPH should be an indication for LT, even if the liver disease is well compensated. Thus, although LT provides benefits for those with PoPH, the question remains whether all those with PoPH should be offered MELD exception points over those with decompensated liver disease or should a more selective approach be considered. The current guidance notes no data to support the concept that PoPH (treated or untreated) should be an indication for LT. Collectively, although PoPH has yet to reach unanimous agreement as an indication for LT, clinicians should strive to optimize PoPH for a qualified candidate and facilitate safe transplants in appropriate candidates, in order to improve the overall outcome.

CLINICS CARE POINTS

- In addition to measuring tricupsid regurgitation velocity, flattening of the interventricular septum, PA diameter >25 mm, IVC diameter > 21 mm with decreased inspiratory collapse all suggest the presence of pulmonary hypertension.
- A normalized PVR is a more reliable marker in predicting perioperative risk for LT than mPAP and exception criteria have been revised to reflect this.

DISCLOSURE

The authors have no relevant commercial or financial conflicts of interest and no funding was received for this article.

REFERENCES

1. Simonneau G, Montani D, Celermajer DS, et al. Haemodynamic definitions and updated clinical classification of pulmonary hypertension. Eur Respir J 2019; 53(1):1801913. https://doi.org/10.1183/13993003.01913-2018.
2. Goldberg DS, Batra S, Sahay S, et al. MELD exceptions for portopulmonary hypertension: current policy and future implementation: transplantation in POPH. Am J Transpl 2014;14(9):2081–7. https://doi.org/10.1111/ajt.12783.
3. Krowka MJ, Swanson KL, Frantz RP, et al. Portopulmonary hypertension: results from a 10-year screening algorithm. Hepatology 2006;44(6):1502–10. https://doi.org/10.1002/hep.21431.
4. Shen M, Zhang F, Zhang X. Pulmonary hypertension in primary biliary cirrhosis: a prospective study in 178 patients. Scand J Gastroenterol 2009;44(2):219–23. https://doi.org/10.1080/00365520802400883.
5. Kawut SM, Krowka MJ, Trotter JF, et al. Clinical risk factors for portopulmonary hypertension. Hepatol Baltim Md 2008;48(1):196–203. https://doi.org/10.1002/hep.22275.
6. Krowka MJ, Miller DP, Barst RJ, et al. Portopulmonary hypertension: a report from the US-based REVEAL Registry. Chest 2012;141(4):906–15. https://doi.org/10.1378/chest.11-0160.
7. Sithamparanathan S, Nair A, Thirugnanasothy L, et al. Survival in portopulmonary hypertension: outcomes of the United Kingdom national pulmonary arterial hypertension registry. J Heart Lung Transpl Off Publ Int Soc Heart Transpl 2017;36(7): 770–9. https://doi.org/10.1016/j.healun.2016.12.014.
8. Lebrec D, Capron JP, Dhumeaux D, et al. Pulmonary hypertension complicating portal hypertension. Am Rev Respir Dis 1979;120(4):849–56. https://doi.org/10.1164/arrd.1979.120.4.849.
9. Robalino BD, Moodie DS. Association between primary pulmonary hypertension and portal hypertension: analysis of its pathophysiology and clinical, laboratory and hemodynamic manifestations. J Am Coll Cardiol 1991;17(2):492–8. https://doi.org/10.1016/s0735-1097(10)80121-4.
10. Medarov BI, Chopra A, Judson MA. Clinical aspects of portopulmonary hypertension. Respir Med 2014;108(7):943–54. https://doi.org/10.1016/j.rmed.2014.04.004.
11. Thomas C, Glinskii V, de Jesus Perez V, et al. Portopulmonary hypertension: from bench to bedside. Front Med 2020;7:569413. https://doi.org/10.3389/fmed.2020.569413.
12. Vallabhajosula S, Radhi S, Cevik C, et al. Hyperthyroidism and pulmonary hypertension: an important association. Am J Med Sci 2011;342(6):507–12. https://doi.org/10.1097/MAJ.0b013e31821790f4.
13. Baeyens N, Bandyopadhyay C, Coon BG, et al. Endothelial fluid shear stress sensing in vascular health and disease. J Clin Invest 2016;126(3):821–8. https://doi.org/10.1172/JCI83083.
14. Garg A, Armstrong WF. Echocardiography in liver transplant candidates. JACC Cardiovasc Imaging 2013;6(1):105–19. https://doi.org/10.1016/j.jcmg.2012.11.002.
15. Taleb M, Khuder S, Tinkel J, et al. The diagnostic accuracy of Doppler echocardiography in assessment of pulmonary artery systolic pressure: a meta-analysis. Echocardiography 2013;30(3):258–65. https://doi.org/10.1111/echo.12061.

16. Silverton N, Meineri M, Djaiani G. The controversy of right ventricular systolic pressure: is it time to abandon the pulmonary artery catheter? Anaesthesia 2015;70(3):241–4. https://doi.org/10.1111/anae.12939.

17. DeMartino ES, Cartin-Ceba R, Findlay JY, et al. Frequency and outcomes of patients with increased mean pulmonary artery pressure at the time of liver transplantation. Transplantation 2017;101(1):101–6. https://doi.org/10.1097/TP.0000000000001517.

18. Rich JD, Shah SJ, Swamy RS, et al. Inaccuracy of Doppler echocardiographic estimates of pulmonary artery pressures in patients with pulmonary hypertension. Chest 2011;139(5):988–93. https://doi.org/10.1378/chest.10-1269.

19. DuBrock HM, Salgia RJ, Sussman NL, et al. Portopulmonary hypertension: a survey of practice patterns and provider attitudes. Transpl Direct 2019;5(6):e456. https://doi.org/10.1097/TXD.0000000000000900.

20. Martin P. Evaluation for liver transplantation in adults. Pract Guideline by AASLD Am Soc Transplant 2013;98. Published online 2013.

21. Krowka MJ, Fallon MB, Kawut SM, et al. International liver transplant society practice guidelines: diagnosis and management of hepatopulmonary syndrome and portopulmonary hypertension. Transplantation 2016;100(7):1440–52. https://doi.org/10.1097/TP.0000000000001229.

22. Galiè N, Humbert M, Vachiery JL, et al. 2015 ESC/ERS guidelines for the diagnosis and treatment of pulmonary hypertension: the joint task force for the diagnosis and treatment of pulmonary hypertension of the European society of cardiology (ESC) and the European respiratory society (ERS)endorsed by: association for European paediatric and congenital cardiology (AEPC), international society for heart and lung transplantation (ISHLT). Eur Respir J 2015;46(4): 903–75. https://doi.org/10.1183/13993003.01032-2015.

23. Krowka M. Pulmonary hemodynamics and perioperative cardiopulmonary-related mortality in patients with portopulmonary hypertension undergoing liver transplantation. Liver Transpl 2000;6(4):443–50. https://doi.org/10.1053/jlts.2000.6356.

24. Aithal GP, Palaniyappan N, China L, et al. Guidelines on the management of ascites in cirrhosis. Gut 2021;70(1):9–29. https://doi.org/10.1136/gutjnl-2020-321790.

25. Provencher S, Herve P, Jais X, et al. Deleterious effects of β-blockers on exercise capacity and hemodynamics in patients with portopulmonary hypertension. Gastroenterology 2006;130(1):120–6. https://doi.org/10.1053/j.gastro.2005.10.013.

26. Peacock A, Ross K. Pulmonary hypertension: a contraindication to the use of -adrenoceptor blocking agents. Thorax 2010;65(5):454–5. https://doi.org/10.1136/thx.2008.111955.

27. Soulaidopoulos S. Pulmonary manifestations of chronic liver disease: a comprehensive review. Ann Gastroenterol 2020. https://doi.org/10.20524/aog.2020.0474.

28. Klinger JR, Kadowitz PJ. The nitric oxide pathway in pulmonary vascular disease. Am J Cardiol 2017;120(8):S71–9. https://doi.org/10.1016/j.amjcard.2017.06.012.

29. Reichenberger F, Voswinckel R, Steveling E, et al. Sildenafil treatment for portopulmonary hypertension. Eur Respir J 2006;28(3):563–7. https://doi.org/10.1183/09031936.06.00030206.

30. Hollatz TJ, Musat A, Westphal S, et al. Treatment with sildenafil and treprostinil allows successful liver transplantation of patients with moderate to severe portopulmonary hypertension. Liver Transpl 2012;18(6):686–95. https://doi.org/10.1002/lt.23407.

31. Cartin-Ceba R, Halank M, Ghofrani H, et al. Riociguat treatment for portopulmonary hypertension: a subgroup analysis from the PATENT-1/-2 studies. Pulm Circ 2018;8(2):1–4. https://doi.org/10.1177/2045894018769305.

32. Hynynen M, Khalil R. The vascular endothelin system in hypertension - recent patents and discoveries. Recent Patents Cardiovasc Drug Discov 2006;1(1): 95–108. https://doi.org/10.2174/157489006775244263.

33. Faisal M, Siddiqi F, Alkaddour A, et al. Effect of PAH specific therapy on pulmonary hemodynamics and six-minute walk distance in portopulmonary hypertension: a systematic review and meta-analysis. Pulm Med 2014;2014:1–7. https://doi.org/10.1155/2014/528783.

34. Current and emerging therapeutic approaches to pulmonary hypertension. Rev Cardiovasc Med 2020;21(2):163. https://doi.org/10.31083/j.rcm.2020.02.597.

35. Sitbon O, Bosch J, Cottreel E, et al. Macitentan for the treatment of portopulmonary hypertension (PORTICO): a multicentre, randomised, double-blind, placebo-controlled, phase 4 trial. Lancet Respir Med 2019;7(7):594–604. https://doi.org/10.1016/S2213-2600(19)30091-8.

36. Sitbon O, Vonk Noordegraaf A. Epoprostenol and pulmonary arterial hypertension: 20 years of clinical experience. Eur Respir Rev 2017;26(143):160055. https://doi.org/10.1183/16000617.0055-2016.

37. Gomberg-Maitland M, Olschewski H. Prostacyclin therapies for the treatment of pulmonary arterial hypertension. Eur Respir J 2008;31(4):891–901. https://doi.org/10.1183/09031936.00097107.

38. DuBrock HM, Goldberg DS, Sussman NL, et al. Predictors of waitlist mortality in portopulmonary hypertension. Transplantation 2017;101(7):1609–15. https://doi.org/10.1097/TP.0000000000001666.

39. Aggarwal M, Li M, Bhardwaj A, et al. Predictors of survival in portopulmonary hypertension: a 20-year experience. Eur J Gastroenterol Hepatol 2022;34(4): 449–56.

40. Jose A, Shah SA, Anwar N, et al. Pulmonary vascular resistance predicts mortality and graft failure in transplantation patients with portopulmonary hypertension. Liver Transpl 2021;27(12):1811–23. https://doi.org/10.1002/lt.26091.

41. DuBrock HM, Runo JR, Sadd CJ, et al. Outcomes of liver transplantation in treated portopulmonary hypertension patients with a mean pulmonary arterial pressure ≥35 mm Hg. Transpl Direct 2020;6(12):e630. https://doi.org/10.1097/TXD.0000000000001085.

42. Cartin-Ceba R, Burger C, Swanson K, et al. Clinical outcomes after liver transplantation in patients with portopulmonary hypertension. Transplantation 2020; 105(10):2283–90.

43. Navarro-Vergara DI, Roldan-Valadez E, Cueto-Robledo G, et al. Portopulmonary hypertension: prevalence, clinical and hemodynamic features. Curr Probl Cardiol 2021;46(3):100747. https://doi.org/10.1016/j.cpcardiol.2020.100747.

44. Enhancements to the national liver review board, OPTN liver and intestinal organ transplantation committee. 2020. Available at: https://optn.transplant.hrsa.gov/media/3927/further_enhancements_nlrb_pc.pdf. Accessed June 1, 2022.

45. Deroo R, Trépo E, Holvoet T, et al. Vasomodulators and liver transplantation for portopulmonary hypertension: evidence from a systematic review and meta-analysis. Hepatology 2020;72(5):1701–16. https://doi.org/10.1002/hep.31164.

46. Barbas AS, Schroder JN, Borle DP, et al. Planned initiation of venoarterial extracorporeal membrane oxygenation prior to liver transplantation in a patient with severe portopulmonary hypertension. Liver Transpl 2021;27(5):760–2. https://doi.org/10.1002/lt.25871.

47. DuBrock HM, Channick RN, Krowka MJ. What's new in the treatment of portopulmonary hypertension? Expert Rev Gastroenterol Hepatol 2015;9(7):983–92. https://doi.org/10.1586/17474124.2015.1035647.

48. Savale L, Sattler C, Coilly A, et al. Long-term outcome in liver transplantation candidates with portopulmonary hypertension: savale et al. Hepatology 2017;65(5):1683–92. https://doi.org/10.1002/hep.28990.
49. Savale L, Guimas M, Ebstein N, et al. Portopulmonary hypertension in the current era of pulmonary hypertension management. J Hepatol 2020;73(1):130–9. https://doi.org/10.1016/j.jhep.2020.02.021.
50. Cartin-Ceba R, Burger C, Swanson K, et al. Clinical outcomes after liver transplantation in patients with portopulmonary hypertension. Transplantation 2021;105(10):2283–90.

Hepatocellular Carcinoma
New Developments

Previn Ganesan, MD, MPH[a],*, Laura M. Kulik, MD[b]

KEYWORDS

- Hepatocellular carcinoma • Cirrhosis • Chemoembolization • Radioembolization
- Liver cancer • Immunotherapy

KEY POINTS

- The epidemiology of hepatocellular carcinoma (HCC) is rapidly evolving, with nonalcoholic fatty liver disease becoming an increasing cause of fibrosis, cirrhosis, and HCC.
- The diagnosis and surveillance of HCC are evolving with the advent of novel biomarkers and development of personalized screening recommendations based on cause of HCC.
- The traditional Barcelona Clinic Liver Cancer staging system has been modified to better represent severity of liver dysfunction and delineate treatment options, especially with the formal introduction of the concept of treatment stage migration.
- There are now advances in curative, noncurative, and combinations of the 2 treatment options. There is increasing research evaluating combinations of therapeutic approaches, including the use of locoregional treatments to "down stage" individuals to reach transplant eligibility.

INTRODUCTION

Hepatocellular carcinoma (HCC) is the fourth leading cause of cancer-related mortality worldwide and a leading cause of death in cirrhosis. The prognosis in HCC is poor, with mortalities approximating incidence rates worldwide.[1,2] The epidemiology of HCC has changed considerably in the past decade. A decrease of viral hepatitis-related cases in certain parts of the world has been offset by an increase in cases related to alcohol and nonalcoholic fatty liver disease (NAFLD) in Western countries. Advancements in the management of HCC, particularly in the advanced stage, have been groundbreaking. Immunotherapy is now being studied in earlier stages of HCC in combination with surgery and locoregional therapy (LRT). This review article provides a summary of recent updates in the epidemiology, diagnosis, staging, and management of HCC.

[a] Northwestern University, 251 East Huron Street, Clarke Conference Room Feinberg Pavilion 13 East, Chicago, IL 60611, USA; [b] Northwestern University, NMH/Arkes Family Pavilion, Suite 1900, 676 North Saint Clair, Chicago, IL 60611, USA
* Corresponding author.
E-mail address: Previn.ganesan@northwestern.edu

Clin Liver Dis 27 (2023) 85–102
https://doi.org/10.1016/j.cld.2022.08.004
1089-3261/23/© 2022 Elsevier Inc. All rights reserved.

Epidemiology

In the United States, the median age of diagnosis is in the sixth decade of life (60–65 among men; 65–69 among women). Generally, HCC is more prevalent among men. There are also numerous observed socioeconomic disparities in HCC incidence, mortality, and survival. HCC incidence and mortality significantly vary by race and ethnicity in the United States, with increased incidence in African American and Hispanic populations. Ongoing research is revealing disparities in HCC by many socioeconomic measures, including neighborhood resources/neighborhood socioeconomic status, insurance type, and geographic location (rural vs urban settings).

HCC occurs in the setting of cirrhosis in approximately 90% of cases. The cause of cirrhosis varies considerably by country. In the United States, the most common causes of cirrhosis leading to HCC are alcohol-related liver disease (ALD), NAFLD or nonalcoholic steatohepatitis (NASH), and viral hepatitis (hepatitis B [HBV] and hepatitis C [HCV]). The most common cause of HCC in the absence of cirrhosis is related to HBV, although there has been an increase in noncirrhotic NAFLD-related HCC.[2] An understanding of risk factors contributing to HCC is essential for prevention efforts, risk stratification, and screening strategies.

DETECTION AND DIAGNOSIS
Surveillance

Surveillance recommendations regarding target population, frequency, and modality of surveillance are complex and dependent on the cost-effectiveness within a targeted population. Early diagnosis with surveillance has consistently demonstrated superior outcomes than symptom-based diagnosis, with respective pooled 3-year survival rates of 50.8% and 27.9%.[3] The American Association for the Study of Liver Diseases (AASLD) will endorse ultrasound (US) + alpha-fetoprotein (AFP) every 6 months in individuals with cirrhosis or certain individuals with HBV (**Box 1**). A meta-analysis reported a higher sensitivity for the detection of early HCC with US + AFP (63%; 95% CI: 48–75%) compared with US alone (53%; 95% CI: 35–70%). Surveillance is not recommended in patients with Child-Pugh C (CP C) or those with comorbid conditions who are not otherwise candidates for liver transplant.[4] Changes in the epidemiology of HCC (ie, increasing incidence of NAFLD), advances in serologic biomarkers, and improvement in imaging modalities may lead to changes in surveillance recommendations in the future.

Moving away from a "one-size-fits-all" approach for HCC surveillance and toward an individualized calculated HCC risk is needed. A personalized approach in patients

---

Box 1
Surveillance tools

AASLD
Annual US + serum AFP in:
- All individuals with cirrhosis
- The following groups with chronic HBV:
  ○ Asian men ≥40 years old
  ○ Asian women ≥50 years old
  ○ Family history of HCC
  ○ Individuals born in Africa ≥20 years old
If unable to adequately assess on US, can pursue multiphase MRI or CT liver.

AASLD guidelines for HCC surveillance in individuals with cirrhosis and/or chronic HBV.

with HCV with sustained virologicresponse (SVR) has been proposed in several risk scores, which may become endorsed if validated in larger cohorts.[5] In addition, such tools may better define the HCC risk in the populations that are not clearly defined (eg, cured HCV with stage 3 fibrosis). Risk scores are also being investigated in other causes of chronic liver disease. A serum protein-based prognostic liver secretome signature (PLSec) comprising 8 proteins has been reported to predict risk of HCC development.[6] This signature combined with AFP (PLSec-AFP) had a superior predictive value than AFP alone. Such an approach could be used to individualize the risk of future HCC to improve cost-effectiveness and focus novel biomarkers (discussed later) on those at the highest risk to detect early HCC.

NAFLD/NASH-induced HCC is increasing owing to the obesity epidemic and is recognized to be the current second most common cause for HCC-related liver transplant. An area of debate is HCC surveillance in noncirrhotic NASH.[7] Although HCC is known to occur in noncirrhotic NASH (20% of NAFLD HCC), screening is not deemed cost-effective and therefore has not been supported by societal guidelines.[8] Recognizing the progression to compensated cirrhosis in NAFLD/NASH to initiate HCC surveillance can be challenging. The SAFE (Steatosis-Associated Fibrosis Estimator) score is a newly devised tool to aid in the detection of stage 2 fibrosis ($\geq$F2 associated with increased morbidity and mortality) among patients with NAFLD, which outperformed both Fibrosis-4 Index (FIB-4)- and NAFLD fibrosis score (NFS). This tool may aid streamlining the most appropriate referrals to liver specialists who have reported higher surveillance rates compared with primary care providers, 73.7% versus 29.5%, respectively.[9] The ability to accurately risk-stratify the plethora of patients with NAFLD (approximately 100 million in the United States) to specialized longitudinal care may lead to timely therapy to prevent development of advanced fibrosis as well as identify those who progress to cirrhosis.

The potential harms of surveillance related to false positive US or AFP levels should be considered when establishing surveillance recommendations. In HCC, the main potential harms are psychological distress, costs of surveillance, and physical harm. A Markov model that considered potential of harm related to additional imaging or biopsy found that US + AFP was the most cost-effective approach over US alone or no surveillance in patients with compensated cirrhosis. A threshold analysis showed that an annual risk of HCC > 0.4% and an adherence of greater than 19.5% were required for US + AFP to be more cost-effective relative to no surveillance.[10]

US may be of limited utility in certain scenarios, including advanced cirrhosis with excessive liver nodularity and/or morbid obesity. One study found that 20% of patients have suboptimal visualization of the liver on US surveillance. Factors significantly associated with US inadequacy include male sex, morbid obesity, fat-associated liver disease, such as ALD and NASH, and advanced liver disease.[11] Such individuals would benefit from cross-sectional imaging. When US is inconclusive, multiphase computed tomographic (CT) scan or MRI should be pursued for surveillance purposes. Although multiphase MRI (liver protocol) may be best for detection of HCC, it is impractical as a surveillance test for all patients. Two studies evaluating MRI demonstrated a pooled sensitivity and specificity of 83.1% (95% CI: 72%–90.5%) and 89.1% (95% CI: 86.5%–91.3%).[12] The PRIUS study reported MRI to be superior to US for early-stage detection of HCC.[13] More recent studies are evaluating abbreviated MRI protocols for screening, which may prove to be more practical as a surveillance method.

Although AFP is used for HCC surveillance, other potential biomarkers are being investigated. Two markers, lens culinaris agglutinin-reactive AFP (AFP-L3) and des-gamma-carboxy prothrombin (DCP), are currently approved for risk-stratification for future development of HCC. GALAD, a composite score of gender, age, AFP, AFP-L3, and DCP, demonstrated sensitivity for any-stage and early-stage detection of greater than 70% and greater than 60% in a multinational cohort of more than 2400 individuals. The Hepatocellular carcinoma Early Detection Strategy study showed that GALAD performed the best for early detection of HCC.[14]

Biomarkers may also function as a prognostic tool. A single-center, prospective study comprising 203 patients (94% received LRT, 18.2% down-staged) with AFP, AFP-L3, and DCP before transplant, was analyzed for post-LT outcomes.[15] Those with an elevated AFP-L3 > 15% and DCP > 7.5% at the time of LT incurred an increased risk of HCC recurrence (HR = 28.4; CI: 6.76–119.9; p< 0.001) post-LT and a significantly lower 3-year overall survival (OS) of 41% compared with 98% in patients without an elevation of AFP-L3 and DCP. Among the 8 recurrences, 63% had elevations in both these biomarkers in contrast to 3.6% not meeting a dual increase in AFP-L3 and DCP. The prognostic role of biomarkers closest to LT was also reported in an earlier retrospective trial.[16] Of note, the cutoff levels for the biomarkers used in these studies were the defined levels to predict risk of developing HCC. Further refinement in the cutoff levels used for LT selection may be warranted.

Possible serum biomarkers that may be of clinical utility in the future include plasma microRNA (miRNA), methylated DNA, circulating tumor DNA (ctDNA) and tumor cells (CTCs), and gene expression profiles (GEPs). MiRNAs are endogenous, short RNA sequences that are involved in posttranscriptional regulation. Certain circulating miRNA levels have been shown to be associated with cirrhosis and HCC in various studies. MiRNA-16, when combined with serologic markers used in the GALAD model, effectively detected 92.4% of HCC cases with 78.5% specificity.[17] Methylated DNA marker (MDM) panels have shown promise in detection of HCC, with some studies demonstrating greater performance than AFP.[18] However, the use of MDM panels needs to be studied in larger cohorts across multiple centers before incorporation into routine surveillance practices. The use of ctDNA and CTCs for surveillance is complex. Because their circulating levels correlate with stage of disease, these tests may not be optimal for early-stage detection. One systematic review evaluating ctDNA and CTCs concluded that these tests will likely be more useful for prognostication and monitoring for recurrence as opposed to initial detection of HCC.[19] Finally, the use of GEPs at the tissue level has identified genetic signatures unique to HCC in smaller sample sizes.[20,21] However, this has yet to be translated to a practical serologic test and has not been evaluated as a screening modality.

Diagnosis

Multiphase CT or MRI with contrast is used for definitive diagnosis of HCC; arterial phase enhancement (APHE); and washout on the portal venous phase. The Liver Reporting and Data System (LIRADS) allows for the classification of liver lesions in cirrhosis in a standardized manner. Multiphase MRI may have higher sensitivity but comparable specificity to CT. Imaging is often sufficient to definitively diagnose HCC (LIRADS-5), eliminating the need for a biopsy for diagnostic purposes. However, when imaging findings are nondiagnostic but highly suspicious for HCC (LIRADS-4), clinicians may repeat an imaging study in 3 months, attempt the alternative imaging modality, or consider pursuing a biopsy for definitive diagnosis. The advantages of CT include shorter duration of examination and lower cost. The disadvantages include exposure to radiation and iodinated contrast. This is especially relevant in individuals with advanced liver disease who can often have concurrent renal dysfunction. The disadvantages of MRI include greater cost, technical complexity, longer examination times, and higher risk of artifact with motion. Of note, the use of gadoxetate disodium, a partially hepatocellular-specific contrast agent for MRI, has not been recommended over traditional extracellular MRI contrast agents. However, some studies suggest that the use of gadoxetate improves sensitivity in detection of small HCC lesions less than 2 cm. For T1 lesions (<2 cm), currently United Network for Organ Sharing (UNOS) requires APHE plus 2 criteria (venous washout, 50% growth over 6 months, or enhancing capsule), whereas LIRADS criteria are less stringent with a diagnosis of HCC made with APHE + venous washout or threshold growth or APHE and 2 criteria. It is anticipated that UNOS will adopt the LIRADS approach in the future for T1 lesions.

STAGING

Staging of HCC is dependent on performance status (PS), degree of liver dysfunction, and traditional TNM staging. The Barcelona Clinic Liver Cancer (BCLC) staging system is recommended by AASLD and European Association for the Study of the Liver (EASL). BCLC classification was recently updated in 2022 to better characterize prognosis and available treatment options. The most notable changes include the following: (1) replacement of CP classification of liver dysfunction with a simplified binary definition of compensated or decompensated liver disease; (2) the introduction of the concept of stage migration; and (3) clarification on decision making in the setting of "evolutionary events" or progression.[22]

Liver function is now characterized as "compensated" or "decompensated." Decompensated liver disease includes the presence of jaundice, ascites, or hepatic encephalopathy, regardless of Model for End-Stage Liver Disease (MELD) or CP classification. Importantly, history of variceal bleeding may represent clinically significant portal hypertension (CSPH) but is not necessarily incorporated into the classification of decompensated or compensated liver disease. Treatment stage migration is the notion that patients may need to be reclassified as more advanced stages because of a variety of factors, even if their overall PS, degree of liver function, and TNM classification remain unchanged. Determining stage migration includes specification of the pattern of progression, considering superior prognosis of enlarging or new intrahepatic lesions compared with new extrahepatic lesions (EHS) or new vascular invasion (VI).

BCLC stage 0 is characterized by a lesion ≤2 cm, without portal vein tumor thrombosis (PVTT) or EHS, compensated liver function, and Eastern Cooperative Oncology Group (ECOG) PS of 0. Expected median survival exceeds 5 years. BCLC stage A also prognosticates survival greater than 5 years. BCLC A consists of a solitary lesion of any size or up to 3 nodules, all ≤3 cm, without vascular or extrahepatic invasion, preserved liver function, and PS of 0. It is important to note that patients who meet criteria for liver transplantation based on tumor burden may be classified as BCLC D because of liver dysfunction or PS. BCLC B is classified as multifocal HCC that exceeds BCLC A, without VI or EHS, preserved liver function, and PS 0. Median survival is 2.5 years for individuals with BCLC stage B HCC. BCLC stage C is defined by VI or EHS, PS ≤ 2, and preserved liver function. Median survival of this stage is approximately 2 years. Finally, BCLC D is characterized by ECOG PS > 2 and impaired liver function. Median survival of individuals with BCLC stage D, if not eligible for orthotopic liver transplantation (OLT), is 3 months.

TREATMENT
Overview

Treatment options are broadly categorized as curative (liver transplantation, resection, or ablation/segmental transarterial radioembolization [TARE]) and noncurative (transarterial chemoembolization [TACE], systemic therapies). When feasible, transplantation is the most definitive treatment option, but organ shortage limits this curative therapy. Systemic therapies are being studied in BCLC A and B to see if this addition to traditional therapy can further improve OS.

Transplantation

Individuals with cirrhosis, significant degree of liver dysfunction, or CSPH, without medical or psychosocial contraindications should pursue liver transplantation. The Milan criteria (MC) have been successfully used as the selection tool for appropriate candidates for OLT based on tumor size and number (**Box 2**). Although this approach has fulfilled an acceptable 5-year OS of greater than 50%,[23] many have thought that the MC are too restrictive and thereby deter OLT in some candidates who would derive long-term OS from transplantation. The field of transplant oncology is evolving because of many concomitant factors: the decrease in patients with HCV requiring OLT because of direct-acting antivirals, living donors, increased use of decreased cardiac death and HCV+ organs, and improvement in available systemic therapies for HCC.

Since the concept of downstaging (DS) to the MC was first published by the University of California, San Francisco (UCSF) group in 2008, additional data support DS as a viable approach to gain access to OLT with excellent post-LT results.[24] Traditionally, the premise of DS is to gain insight into the biological activity of tumors exceeding the MC based on the response to LRT. A key component of the UCSF-DS protocol has been an upper tumor burden: 1 lesion greater than 5 cm and ≤8 cm, 2 or 3 lesions each ≤5 cm and total diameter of all lesions ≤8 cm, 4 or 5 lesions each ≤3 cm and total diameter of all lesions ≤8 cm, and absence of VI/EHS. UCSF-DS criteria have been synonymous with UNOS-DS since acceptance of DS into UNOS guidelines.

A subsequent study compared UCSF-DS with an AC-DS, which allowed any tumor size, number, or diameter without VI/EHS.[25] A difference between these 2 cohorts included a longer minimal observation period from successful DS to the MC to OLT in the AC-DS group (6 months) compared with the USCF-DS group, 3 months. In addition, the development of any new lesion in the AC-DS group was criteria for exclusion for OLT. Among the 74 patients that were treated in the AC-DS group, 48 (64.8%) achieved DS of which 10 (13.5%) underwent OLT and 3 developed recurrent HCC after a median of 21 months posttransplant. The only factor that was associated with successful DS in the AC-DS group was a decrease after LRT in the sum of the largest lesion + number of tumors. The AC-DS group was more likely to drop out at 1 and 3 years (53.5% and 80.0%) compared with the UCSF-DS group (25.0% and

---

Box 2
Milan criteria and eligibility for downstaging

Milan criteria
- 1 lesion ≥2 cm and ≤5 cm or
- Up to 3 lesions, each ≥1 cm and ≤3 cm and
- No vascular invasion or extrahepatic spread

UNOS/UCSF eligibility for downstaging:
- 1 lesion >5 cm ≤ 8 cm or
- 2–3 lesions >3 cm and ≤5 cm, total tumor diameter ≤8 cm
- 4–5 lesions each ≤3 cm, total tumor diameter ≤8 cm

Criteria for liver transplant eligibility in patients with HCC followed by criteria that is acceptable for attempting down-staging to reach transplant eligibility.

36.1%). In addition to sum of largest lesion and tumor number, CP class B/C was an independent predictor of dropout. Furthermore, the post 5-year OLT survival was lower in the AC-DS group (21.1%) compared with UCSF-DS (56.0%). The overall inferior rate of successful DS, OS post-OLT, and higher dropout rates led the authors to conclude that an upper limit of tumor burden is required for optimal outcomes (see **Box 2**).

A national study comprising 3819 transplants with an MELD upgrade that occurred between 2012 and 2015 explored the outcome of 3 groups: MC (N = 3276), UNOS-DS (N = 422), and AC-DS (N = 121).[26] Those who underwent OLT among AC-DC had significantly lower 3-year OS (71.4%) compared with the MC group (83.2%). From an HCC perspective, the AC-DS cohort had worse 3-year HCC recurrence rates (16.7% vs 12.8% vs 6.9%), higher rates of VI on explant (23.7% vs 16.9% vs 14.2%), and higher explant pathology (40.5% vs 32.5% vs 14.2%) compared with UNOS-DS and MC, respectively. Key findings of this study showed the importance of tumor biology in the selection of candidates for LT after DS to the MC. The first was that the median wait time defined as short (2.6 months) was a significant predictor of death post-LT in those who required DS relative to regions with mid (6.5 months) and long (12.8 months) waiting times (HR, 3.07; CI: 1.41–6.67). An AFP > 100 ng/mL versus less than 20 ng/mL closest to LT was also an independent predictor of mortality post-LT in the UNOS-DS and AC-DS groups, with a 3-year OS of 60% and recurrence rate of 25% in the DS groups when the AFP > 100 ng/mL. Specifically in the AC-DS group, the 3-year OS dropped to 50% if the AFP was greater than 20 ng/mL. The interplay of AFP and tumor burden noted in this study is in line with Metroticket 2.0, which considers AFP level, tumor size, and number to predict HCC-specific 5-year OS post-LT.[27]

Additional valuable data on DS to LT come from a prospective trial for the Multicenter Evaluation of the Reduction in Tumor Size before Liver Transplantation Consortium,[28] which recruited patients from 7 centers in the United States from 4 different regions from 2016 to 2019. All 209 enrolled patients fulfilled the UNOS-DS criteria. DS was successful in 83% of patients. Although patients were more likely to be treated with TACE, there was no significant difference in the success of DS between TACE (N = 132) and TARE (N = 62). DS was successful in 83% of patients. The dropout rate was 37%, including the 35 patients that were never downstaged and 40 patients that progressed after initial DS. The only factor that predicted dropout was a pretreatment AFP-L3 $\geq$ 10%. Although this supports the validity of DS with a 3-year OS of 72% from the receipt of initial LRT, it did have a cautionary finding of 43% of patients exceeding the MC on explant. The risk of understaging was associated with the number of tumors plus the largest tumor diameter on the last pre-LT scan. These results support using LRT for the goal of complete response (CR) to minimize the risk of understaging.

A randomized controlled trial (RCT) called the XXL trial from 4 centers in Italy randomized patients exceeding the MC (without PVTT/EHS) to LT versus continued LRT.[29] Patients who were BCLC B were recruited using the Metroticket 2.0 calculator and those with a predicted 5-year OS of at least 50% using baseline tumor size, number, and AFP level were eligible. A total of 74 patients were enrolled, of which 54 met criteria for successful DS using LRT, surgery, or systemic therapy (limited to sorafenib) per each center's multidisciplinary team (MDT). They were then randomized after a 3-month observation period to continued LRT and systemic therapy at the time of tumor progression versus listing for LT. A total of 45 patients were randomized in a 1:1 fashion to LT arm (n = 23) or to the control group (n = 22); 21 underwent LT (2 refused transplant). This study was intended to enroll 260 subjects; however, the trial was stopped prematurely reflecting the challenges of conducting an RCT that involves

LT. Nonetheless, transplantation resulted in superior 5-year OS of 77.5% (95% CI: 61.9–97.1) compared with the nontransplant group (31.2%; 95% CI: 16.6–58.5). Some of the limitations of the trial included a long time to reach DS criteria (18 months), which was not the traditional MC. The accompanying editorial to this trial suggested that the more ideal trial design would have been a centralized MDT, with successful DS defined as CR and a longer period of observation before randomization (6 months is required by UNOS post-DS to MC) and inclusion of explant pathology in the analysis.[30] To date, this is the only study that has included LT in a randomized trial. The results are encouraging and reinforce the role of DS to LT. It remains to be seen how the deprioritization of the HCC MELD to the median MELD score at transplant for a given transplant referral region minus 3 points will impact dropout in patients who have been successfully DS.

The presence of PVVT has been considered an absolute contraindication for LT because of the high rate of HCC recurrence post-LT. UNOS recently has clarified that careful selection of some patients with branch PVVT who have had achieved prolonged (minimum of 12 months) treatment response may be considered for LT.

A multicenter, international retrospective trial reported the outcomes of 30 patients with PVTT,[31] excluding main PVTT (pV4) who underwent LT after LRT. The 5-year OS was 60%. The investigators identified that the pre-LT AFP was an independent predictor of HCC recurrence post-LT with the ideal AFP cutoff being less than 10 ng/mL. An AFP < 10 ng/mL was associated with a recurrence rate of 11% compared with 50% in those with an AFP > 10 ng/mL ($P = .019$). Explant findings that significantly increased the chance of HCC recurrence included the presence of viable HCC, number of viable tumors, satellite nodules, and greater than MC.

A pilot study from Italy enrolled 17 patients with PVTT (Vp1, n = 3; Vp2, n = 5; Vp3, n = 9) attempted to DS with TARE and listed 6 patients for OLT post-Y90 after meeting the following criteria: tumor burden fulfilled MC, a sustained response greater than 6 months of no enhancement in the PVTT, and AFP < 100 ng/mL.[32] Five patients underwent OLT, of which 3 developed HCC recurrence. Although there was no significant difference in characteristics between the nontransplanted and transplanted patients, there was a higher portion of patients in the nontransplant group with an AFP > 100 ng/mL (41.7% vs 0%). The 1 patient who died of progressive HCC post-LT had an AFP > 10 ng/mL (19 ng/mL) before transplant, which emphasizes the role of tumor biology in DS. The other 2 patients with HCC recurrence occurred in the lung treated with resection, highlighting the important role of resection when feasible for HCC recurrence post-LT to attain long-term OS.

The field of transplant oncology is rapidly evolving as the treatment options, particularly immunotherapy, have expanded. The use of immune checkpoint inhibitors (ICIs) before LT had been considered a contraindication because of fear of graft dysfunction/loss. A case report of a patient who had received Nivolumab for 2 years before LT (8 days after the last dose) died 6 days post-LT owing to hepatic necrosis despite aggressive therapy for acute cellular rejection that supported this theoretical concern. However, subsequent small retrospective series have not seen graft loss.[33–35] UNOS has put forth that, although data on the use of immunotherapy to bridge or DS to LT are preliminary, receipt of ICI alone is not a contraindication to receive an HCC MELD upgrade. Ongoing trials in China, PLENTY202001 and DULECT2020-1, are exploring the role of combination therapy with ICI plus TKI (**Table 1**). It is hoped that such trials will address several critical questions, such as: (1) Does response to combination therapy allow decrease post-LT HCC recurrence in those exceeding the MC? (2) Do ICIs increase risk of graft dysfunction? (3) What is the appropriate time period to stop ICIs

Table 1
Current trials evaluating immune checkpoint inhibitors in combination with tyrosine kinase inhibitors

	PLENTY202001 NCT04425226 (N = 192)	Dulect2020-1 NCT04443322 (N = 20)
Study design	RCT: Lenvatinib + pembrolizumab vs no intervention	Prospective open label: Durvalumab + lenvatinib
Population	HCC > MC before LT	Locally advanced HCC before LT
Primary endpoint	Recurrence-free survival up to 4 years	Recurrence-free survival up to 4 y
Duration of therapy	• Pembrolizumab until 42 days before LT or unacceptable toxicity • LEN until 7 days before LT	• Durva until 42 d before LT or unacceptable toxicity • LEN until 7 days before LT

before LT and observe for PD off ICI as well as minimize risk of ACR? (4) Are there biomarkers to determine the tumor response and immune system degree of activation?

Resection

Resection is recommended for early-stage HCC without VI. In select patient groups, outcomes with resection are comparable to those with transplant. Resection is equivalent to ablation for tumors ≤2 cm, so radiofrequency (RFA) or microwave ablation (MWA) should be pursued for smaller tumors. There is also mounting evidence that MWA may be appropriate for tumors up to 4 cm. For larger tumors, resection is preferred. Although not performed frequently in the United States, resection in the setting of low-grade VI or portal vein tumor thrombus (PVTT) is used in certain countries with successful outcomes.[36]

Multiple studies are evaluating the use of neoadjuvant therapies before resection. Notable neoadjuvant modalities include TACE, TARE, and systemic therapies. TACE before resection has been associated with worse survival, increased morbidity, and greater utilization of medical resources in multiple earlier studies because of delay to resection and progressive disease.[37,38] TARE is safe and effective in bridging patients with initially unresectable HCC to resection or transplant.[39] However, there have been no randomized trials evaluating its role as standard neoadjuvant therapy. The safety and tolerability of neoadjuvant immunotherapy are being investigated across multiple phase 2 trials. Kaseb, Pinato, and colleagues[40–42] report a 25% complete pathologic response in a small cohort of patients who were randomized to nivolumab or combination ipilimumab/nivolumab perioperatively. A recent phase 3 multicenter RCT in China showed significantly improved OS and progression-free survival (PFS) with neoadjuvant transarterial FOLFOX chemotherapy compared with standard resection (3-year OS 63.5% vs 46.3%; $P = .016$).[43] The risk of recurrence after resection depends on tumor differentiation, presence of microvascular invasion, and tumor size or burden. Annual recurrence rate after resection is estimated to be ≥10%, with 5-year recurrence risk approaching 70% to 80%.[44] Approximately 66% of recurrence events will occur within the first 2 years following resection, and it remains to be seen if immunotherapy can decrease, delay, or impact the pattern of recurrence.

Locoregional Therapies

Uses

LRTs encompass a wide variety of techniques, some of which are used with curative intent. Broadly, ablative techniques are curative therapies used for smaller tumors.

Embolization techniques are used for relatively advanced stages (BCLC B) to prolong survival. Embolization can also be used as a "bridge" to transplant (prevent progression of HCC beyond MC) or to downstage HCC to within MC. There are multiple ongoing RCTs evaluating combinations of LRTs and systemic therapies, in either the neoadjuvant or the adjuvant setting.

Ablation

Ablation is an appropriate therapeutic approach for smaller tumors, ideally less than 3 to 4 cm. Thermal ablation includes the use of microwaves, radiofrequency, cryotherapy, and laser interstitial thermal therapy (LITT). Other ablative techniques incorporate the use of alcohol or electroporation. At this time, MWA and RFA are most common. Multiple studies have shown comparable efficacy between MWA and RFA, but more recent studies suggest improved tumor control with MWA.[45,46] Important considerations aside from tumor size include location of the tumor, risk of tumor seeding, and the inability to obtain tumor samples to be evaluated by a pathologist. Tumors should be more centrally located with a sufficient margin of normal liver tissue to ensure successful ablation. Generally, the use of ablative techniques should achieve a 10-mm margin surrounding the tumor. This is to maximize removal of any microsatellite lesions, which have been shown to predominantly occur within 10 mm of HCC lesions. RFA and MWA have been shown to be comparable to resection for smaller tumors (<2 cm) and should be the first-line approach, consistent with AASLD, EASL, and APASL.[47] Median OS with RFA is 60 months, with a 5-year relative risk of 50% to 70%.[48] A recent meta-analysis that compared local ablative techniques to surgical resection showed similar OS but improved RFS and local recurrence rates with resection (HR, 0.75; 95% CI: 0.65–0.96). Resection led to improved OS and RFS compared with MWA and RFA + TACE.[49] The major complications of ablative techniques include infection or abscess formation, excessive bleeding, liver failure, and tumor seeding. Predictors of increased risk of complication include advanced liver disease, increased tumor size, and increased ablation zone size.[50]

Cryoablation, electroporation, and LITT are less frequently used. Alcohol ablation should no longer be used, as RFA and MWA are known to be superior in terms of tumor response and survival. Cryoablation has been shown to be similarly efficacious to and possibly safer than RFA and MWA in certain settings.[51,52] However, limited studies evaluating this technique prevent its widespread adoption in the United States. Electroporation may be of use when tumors are in unfavorable locations (ie, near vasculature or biliary ducts). The nature of electroporation, which involves delivery of a high-voltage current to target tissue, allows more precise targeting of tumor and less off-target effects to healthy tissues.[50]

Some studies have suggested increased benefit when RFA is combined with chemoembolization, intratumoral iodine, or intravenous liposomal doxorubicin. One study reported superior OS with the combination of TACE and RFA compared with RFA alone in HCC tumors less than 7 cm.[53] Another study demonstrated improved survival with combination RFA and intratumoral iodine-125 seed implantation compared with RFA alone.[54] There may be a role for combination immunotherapy, tyrosine kinase inhibitors (TKIs), and anti-VEGF therapies with ablative techniques. Ablation has been shown to increase recruitment of cytotoxic T cells to the tumor microenvironment. Increased cytotoxic T-cell activity by immune checkpoint inhibition may prove to be complementary to increased T-cell recruitment observed with ablation. Although multiple studies have demonstrated improved survival with adjuvant or neoadjuvant therapies, no multimodal approach has accumulated enough evidence to be incorporated into AASLD recommendations at this time.

A novel ablative technique in development is phototherapy. Photodynamic and photothermal therapies use certain light wavelengths to induce physical and chemical changes that result in tumor death. Challenges to this potential technique include limited delivery of certain light wavelengths percutaneously. Hence, various technologies to aid in local delivery of phototherapy are being developed. Multiple groups have reported effective nanoparticle-based phototherapeutics to ablate orthotopic HCC in mouse models.[55,56]

Embolization

There are multiple embolization techniques, including transarterial bland embolization (TAE), TACE, drug-eluting bead TACE (DEB-TACE), and TARE. TAE consists of bland embolization of arteries supplying a tumor without concurrent administration of any antitumoral agents. This is not commonly performed since the advent of more advanced techniques (eg, TACE, TARE).

Transarterial chemoembolization

TACE involves the administration of lipiodol-based chemotherapeutics before embolization of arterial vessels feeding a tumor. DEB-TACE replaces the lipiodol-based antitumoral agent with DEB carrying an antitumoral agent. This has been shown to increase local delivery of antitumoral agents and decrease systemic exposure. TACE, which is regarded as equivalent to DEB-TACE, is the current standard of care for intermediate stage HCC (BCLC B).[50] TACE can be used to promote survival, as a bridge to transplant, or for DS. Expected survival with TACE in appropriately selected patients is 20 to 37 months, with a median survival of 30 months. A notable challenge with TACE and other LRTs is the identification of patients who would be able to safely tolerate and derive significant benefit from TACE. BCLC B within the new staging system should better identify individuals who will benefit from TACE.

Transarterial radioembolization

TARE was granted approval for the treatment of HCC based on the Local radioEmbolization using Glass Microspheres for the Assessment of Tumor Control with Y-90 (LEGACY) study.[57] This was a multicenter, single-arm retrospective study in the United States of 162 patients with a single lesion greater than 2 cm and ≤8 cm, CP A, BCLC A or C (based on PS of 1) who were treated with TARE using an ablative dose of radiation (>190 Gy delivered to the targeted lesion). The primary outcomes were objective response rate (ORR) and duration of response (DoR) based on local mRECIST using blinded, independent central review. ORR was seen in 72.6% and DoR ≥ 6 months was seen in 76.1% of patients. The 3-year OS for the entire cohort was 86.6%, which increased to 93.1% among the 45 patients that subsequently had adjuvant therapy with hepatic resection (N = 11) or transplantation (N = 34) after Y90. Of note, the updated BCLC staging system now lists TARE as a potential therapy in early HCC not eligible for or failure after ablation, resection, or transplantation.

The DOSIPHERE trial was an RCT in France comparing the response rate in personalized dosimetry (PD; >205 Gy to the targeted tumor) with standard dosimetry (SD; 120 ± 20 Gy) in patients treated with glass microspheres.[58] In contrast to the LEGACY study, which excluded PV involvement, the majority of patients in this RCT had PVTT, and the median size of the treated lesion was up 10 to 11 cm compared with 2.7 cm in the LEGACY study. There was a significant improvement in response rate in those treated with PD (76.6%) compared with SD (22.2%), which led to significant improvement in the median OS between the 2 groups: 26.6 months (PD) versus 10.7 months (SD) (HR = 0.421; 95% CI: 0.215–0.826). In addition, the use of boosted radiation in the PD translated to a higher rate of secondary surgery (resection or OLT) 35%

compared with 3.5% in SD ($P = .0024$). Among the patients that had explant data, there was complete pathologic necrosis when segmental dose exceeded 400 Gy. These results challenge the validity of the negative RCTs that compared Y90 with sorafenib; none of these trials employed PD and had median OS in the Y90-treated group, similar to the SD arm in DOSIPHERE.

The TRACE trial, a multicenter RCT comparing glass microspheres to DEB-TACE, reported improved TTP,[59] the primary endpoint (17.1 vs. 9.5 months; $P = .002$) and OS (30.2 vs 15.6 months; $P = .06$) in the TARE group at the interim analysis, leading to early termination of this trial. The safety profile between the 2 forms of intra-arterial therapy was equivalent. PREMEIRE, an earlier RCT comparing Y90 to TACE, demonstrated similar results. Of note, boosted radiation using personalized dosimetry was not used in these RCTs and therefore may have underestimated the benefit seen with TARE. One form of intra-arterial therapy over the other is often driven by center experience and not endorsed by guidelines.

Stereotactic body radiation therapy

The role of stereotactic body radiation therapy (SBRT) in the management of HCC has not been established. SBRT is a form of external beam radiation therapy that allows high doses of radiation to be precisely delivered to tumors in a small number of fractions. RFA was reported to improve survival compared with SBRT in a meta-analysis.[60] Other retrospective analyses have shown similar rates of tumor control with SBRT compared with RFA or TACE. For certain tumor sizes, SBRT may be comparable to TACE in establishing tumor control and OS. The use of SBRT in more advanced HCC may improve survival when compared with sorafenib alone.[50,61] A pivotal prospective study established the role of SBRT in conjunction with embolization techniques to downstage patients with HCC and PVTT as a bridge to successful living donor transplantation.[62] Their findings suggest effective DS as evidenced by elimination of PVTT fluorodeoxyglucose avidity after SBRT and/or radioembolization.

Embolization + systemics

Several RCTs combining systemic therapy with intra-arterial techniques have not shown a benefit to support this practice. Specifically, the use of TACE + TKIs has failed to improve outcomes compared with TACE alone. Challenges in trial design and variability of embolization techniques have been posed as explanations for negative results. TACTICS, a trial in Japan, took a unique approach in its trial design and did not consider new hepatic lesions as progressive disease. Patients were continued in their respective treatment arm until development of untreatable, unTACEable progression, CP C, or VI/EHS. PFS, one of the primary endpoints, was significantly improved with TACE + sorafenib compared with TACE (22.8 vs 13.5 months; HR = 0.661; $P = .02$); however, OS did not meet its endpoint (36.2 vs. 30.8 months; $P = .40$).[63]

Based on data to support that LRT can provide a synergistic effect with immunotherapies, several trials are currently examining the safety and efficacy of TACE plus a single-agent ICI as well as TACE with combination systemic therapy including doublets of ICIs, ICI + TKI, and ICI + bevacizumab. One study is looking at TACE + cabozantinib with ipilimumab/nivolumab in a single-center, single-arm phase 2 study (NCT04472767). CheckMate 74W is a global phase 3 trial in patients with HCC that exceeds the MC but within up to 7 criteria randomized to 3 arms in a 1:1:1 fashion: NIVO + IPI + TACE (arm A), NIVO + IPI placebo + TACE (arm B), or NIVO placebo + IPI placebo + TACE (arm C) (NCT04340193). Similar studies are also being conducted using TARE + ICIs compared with TARE alone (NCT05063565). If positive, the management of intermediate HCC could become transformed. The more agents used in combination must be balanced with the risk of increased adverse events and reduced tolerability even in well compensated cirrhosis.

Intra-arterial therapies combined with systemic therapy are also being explored in BCLC C. The LAUNCH study conducted in China with predominately HBV-induced HCC reached its primary endpoint of improved OS associated with lenvatinib + TACE compared with lenvatinib alone (17.8 vs 11.5 months; HR, 0.45; P ≤.001) in CP A patients with advanced HCC.[64] PFS was also superior, being 10.6 months with combination therapy compared with 6.4 months in lenvatinib monotherapy (HR, 0.43; P<.001). Although this study strengthens the potential role of LRT combined with systemic therapy, it is not clear that these results are translatable to a US population that has less HBV.

Systemic Therapies

After the approval of sorafenib in 2007 for advanced HCC, another systemic agent was not approved for over a decade. Over the last few years, the landscape for BCLC C has rapidly expanded. Although there has been approval of several single agents in first (lenvatinib) and second line (regorefenib, cabozantinib, ramucirumab, pembrolizumab), the era of combination therapy has demonstrated the most promising results. In 2019, the IMBRAVE 150 showed that the combination of atezolizumab/bevacizumab met its dual primary endpoint of significant improvement in OS and PFS compared with sorafenib (OS: 19.2 vs 13.2; PFS: 6.9 vs 4.2). This has led to this combination becoming the preferred primary therapy in advanced HCC. The HIMALAYA trial was presented at the American Society of Clinical Oncology Gastroenterology meeting in 2022. The combination of tremelimumab 300 mg, a CTLA 4 inhibitor × 1 + durvalumab 1500 mg × every 4 weeks, a PDL-1 inhibitor, outperformed sorafenib when it met the primary endpoint (OS: 16.4 vs 13.4 months; HR = 0.78; 95% CI: 0.65–0.92). However, PFS, the secondary endpoint, was comparable between the 2 groups (3.75 vs 4.07 months; HR = 0.86; 95% CI: 0.73–1.03). This is the first RCT in HCC to show significantly improved OS without improved PFS. Of note, an EGD before enrollment was not mandated. It is anticipated that tremelimumab plus durvalumab will become the next Food and Drug Adminstration–approved therapy in unresectable HCC. COSMIC 312, a phase 3 trial that looked at combination therapy with cabozantinib plus atezolizumab compared with sorafenib, failed to show a significant difference in OS despite a significant improved PFS in the combination group. Another phase 3 trial, CheckMate 9DW, is awaiting readout in first-line therapy comparing nivolumab plus ipilimumab (currently approved in the second line) to monotherapy LEN or sorafenib in BCLC C (NCT04039607).

TKIs have been postulated to decrease tumor resistance to immunotherapy and are being studied in combination with immunotherapy agents. A phase 1b trial reported a promising median OS of 22.0 months in patients with unresectable HCC treated with lenvatinib plus pembrolizumab.[65] A real world retrospective study examined 123 patients treated with LEN + pembrolizumab compared with LEN monotherapy and showed improved ORR, disease control rate, and PFS with combination therapy.[66] The results of LEAP-002, a phase 3 RCT of lenvatinib plus pembrolizumab, compared with lenvatinib monotherapy are anxiously awaited (NCT03713593). Overall, the role of TKIs as monotherapy may begin to decline; they remain an important therapeutic option for those who are ineligible for immunotherapy and may prove to be an efficacious adjunct to immunotherapy.

An unmet need in the systemic space is among those with decompensated cirrhosis, as the registration trials leading to approval of these agents were limited to CP A patients. Real world data sets in CP B patients treated with atezolizumab/

bevacizumab have been reported. D'Alessio and colleagues[67] conducted a retrospective study from 11 centers in UK/Europe/Asia January 2019 to January 2021 of 202 patients treated with atezolizumab/bevacizumab of which 48 patients were CP B (7–9) at the initiation of therapy. There was no significant difference in safety between CP A and B. EGD data were available in 53% of patients. Interestingly, there was no association with the initial size of esophageal varices or CP classification with risk of EV bleed, which occurred in 14% of patients.

SUMMARY

In this review, the authors summarize the current state of epidemiology, detection, diagnosis, and treatment of HCC. The epidemiology and management of HCC have undergone a significant transformation in the past decade. The cause of HCC is increasingly attributable to metabolic disorders and less to viral hepatitis as HBV and HCV treatment becomes more effective and available. The surveillance and diagnosis of HCC are evolving with the advent of novel biomarkers and repurposing existing surveillance tools. However, equally important is tailored risk-stratification of patients and understanding subgroups who would benefit from particular surveillance and treatment strategies. The new BCLC staging system, which has been updated with consideration of novel treatment strategies, should help clarify optimal treatment plans. The therapeutic landscape for HCC is vast and exponentially growing. There have been tremendous advancements in expanding transplant eligibility with the acceptance of the concept of "downstaging." More studies involving LRTs have allowed for improved identification of eligible candidates and an understanding of the risk/benefit profiles of these interventions. Immunotherapy has transformed the treatment of every stage of HCC and has potential to complement nearly every other therapeutic approach. These therapeutic innovations are accompanied by the challenge of rigorous head-to-head comparisons of various treatment strategies. Continued international collaboration will be key to understanding how to best manage HCC.

CLINICS CARE POINTS

- The adoption of the novel Barcelona Clinic Liver Cancer staging system is essential to navigating the numerous treatment options for hepatocellular carcinoma.
- Certain patients, as outlined by the United Network for Organ Sharing/UCSF down-staging criteria, may initially be beyond the Milan criteria but able to be down staged to transplant eligibility with locoregional therapy.
- Treatment stage migration is distinct from down-staging and represents the escalation to a later stage based on multiple characteristics.
- There are increasing indications for immunotherapy in hepatocellular carcinoma, with atezolizumab and bevacizumab becoming the preferred first-line therapy in eligible patients. Ongoing research is evaluating the use of immunotherapy in conjunction with definitive and locoregional therapies.

REFERENCES

1. McGlynn KA, Petrick JL, El-Serag HB. Epidemiology of hepatocellular carcinoma. Hepatology 2021;73(S1):4–13.
2. Mittal S, El-Serag HB, Sada YH, et al. Hepatocellular carcinoma in the absence of cirrhosis in United States veterans is associated with nonalcoholic fatty liver disease. Clin Gastroenterol Hepatol 2016;14(1):124–31.e1.

3. Kanwal F, Singal AG. Surveillance for hepatocellular carcinoma: current best practice and future direction. Gastroenterology 2019;157(1):54–64.

4. Tzartzeva K, Obi J, Rich NE, et al. Surveillance imaging and alpha fetoprotein for early detection of hepatocellular carcinoma in patients with cirrhosis: a meta-analysis. Gastroenterology 2018;154(6):1706–18.e1.

5. Semmler G, Mandorfer M. Reply to: 'Risk stratification of hepatocellular carcinoma after hepatitis C virus eradication in patients with compensated advanced chronic liver disease in Japan'. J Hepatol 2022. https://doi.org/10.1016/j.jhep.2022.04.031.

6. Fujiwara N, Kobayashi M, Fobar AJ, et al. A blood-based prognostic liver secretome signature and long-term hepatocellular carcinoma risk in advanced liver fibrosis. Med (N Y). 2021;2(7):836–50.e10.

7. Wong RJ, Cheung R, Ahmed A. Nonalcoholic steatohepatitis is the most rapidly growing indication for liver transplantation in patients with hepatocellular carcinoma in the U.S. Hepatology 2014;59(6):2188–95.

8. Kanwal F, Kramer JR, Mapakshi S, et al. Risk of hepatocellular cancer in patients with non-alcoholic fatty liver disease. Gastroenterology 2018;155(6):1828–37.e2.

9. Wolf E, Rich NE, Marrero JA, et al. Use of hepatocellular carcinoma surveillance in patients with cirrhosis: a systematic review and meta-analysis. Hepatology 2021;73(2):713–25.

10. Parikh ND, Singal AG, Hutton DW, et al. Cost-effectiveness of hepatocellular carcinoma surveillance: an assessment of benefits and harms. Am J Gastroenterol 2020;115(10):1642–9.

11. Simmons O, Fetzer DT, Yokoo T, et al. Predictors of adequate ultrasound quality for hepatocellular carcinoma surveillance in patients with cirrhosis. Aliment Pharmacol Ther 2017;45(1):169–77.

12. Roberts LR, Sirlin CB, Zaiem F, et al. Imaging for the diagnosis of hepatocellular carcinoma: a systematic review and meta-analysis. Hepatology 2018;67(1):401–21.

13. Kim SY, An J, Lim YS, et al. MRI with liver-specific contrast for surveillance of patients with cirrhosis at high risk of hepatocellular carcinoma. JAMA Oncol 2017;3(4):456–63.

14. Marrero J.A., Parikh N.D., Roberts L.R., et al., GALAD score improves early detection of HCC prior to the diagnosis of HCC: a phase 3 biomarker validation study. American Association for the Study of the Liver. The Liver Meeting 2021.

15. Kotwani P, Chan W, Yao F, et al. DCP and AFP-L3 are complementary to AFP in predicting high-risk explant features: results of a prospective study. Clin Gastroenterol Hepatol 2022;20(3):701–3.e2.

16. Chaiteerakij R, Zhang X, Addissie BD, et al. Combinations of biomarkers and Milan criteria for predicting hepatocellular carcinoma recurrence after liver transplantation. Liver Transpl 2015;21(5):599–606.

17. Borel F, Konstantinova P, Jansen PL. Diagnostic and therapeutic potential of miRNA signatures in patients with hepatocellular carcinoma. J Hepatol 2012;56(6):1371–83.

18. Kisiel JB, Dukek BA, VSRK R, et al. Hepatocellular carcinoma detection by plasma methylated DNA: discovery, phase I pilot, and phase II clinical validation. Hepatology 2019;69(3):1180–92.

19. Chen VL, Xu D, Wicha MS, et al. Utility of liquid biopsy analysis in detection of hepatocellular carcinoma, determination of prognosis, and disease monitoring: a systematic review. Clin Gastroenterol Hepatol 2020;18(13):2879–902.e9.

20. Chen J, Zaidi S, Rao S, et al. Analysis of genomes and transcriptomes of hepatocellular carcinomas identifies mutations and gene expression changes in the transforming growth factor-β pathway. Gastroenterology 2018;154(1):195–210.

21. Hoshida Y, Villanueva A, Kobayashi M, et al. Gene expression in fixed tissues and outcome in hepatocellular carcinoma. N Engl J Med 2008;359(19):1995–2004.

22. Reig M, Forner A, Rimola J, et al. BCLC strategy for prognosis prediction and treatment recommendation: the 2022 update. J Hepatol 2022;76(3):681–93.

23. Bruix J, Fuster J, Llovet JM. Liver transplantation for hepatocellular carcinoma: foucault pendulum versus evidence-based decision. Liver Transpl 2003;9(7):700–2.

24. Yao FY, Kerlan RK Jr, Hirose R, et al. Excellent outcome following down-staging of hepatocellular carcinoma prior to liver transplantation: an intention-to-treat analysis. Hepatology 2008;48(3):819–27.

25. Sinha J, Mehta N, Dodge JL, et al. Are there upper limits in tumor burden for down-staging of hepatocellular carcinoma to liver transplant? Analysis of the all-comers protocol. Hepatology 2019;70(4):1185–96.

26. Mehta N, Dodge JL, Grab JD, et al. National experience on down-staging of hepatocellular carcinoma before liver transplant: influence of tumor burden, alpha-fetoprotein, and wait time. Hepatology 2020;71(3):943–54.

27. Mazzaferro V, Sposito C, Zhou J, et al. Metroticket 2.0 model for analysis of competing risks of death after liver transplantation for hepatocellular carcinoma. Gastroenterology 2018;154(1):128–39.

28. Mehta N, Frenette C, Tabrizian P, et al. Downstaging outcomes for hepatocellular carcinoma: results from the multicenter evaluation of reduction in tumor size before liver transplantation (MERITS-LT) consortium. Gastroenterology 2021;161(5):1502–12.

29. Mazzaferro V, Citterio D, Bhoori S, et al. Liver transplantation in hepatocellular carcinoma after tumour downstaging (XXL): a randomised, controlled, phase 2b/3 trial. Lancet Oncol 2020;21(7):947–56.

30. Ferrer-Fàbrega J, Forner A. Is downstaging a reliable strategy for expanding criteria for liver transplantation in hepatocellular carcinoma? Lancet Oncol 2020;21(7):867–9.

31. Assalino M, Terraz S, Grat M, et al. Liver transplantation for hepatocellular carcinoma after successful treatment of macrovascular invasion – a multi-center retrospective cohort study. Transpl Int 2020;33(5):567–75.

32. Serenari M, Cappelli A, Cucchetti A, et al. Deceased donor liver transplantation after radioembolization for hepatocellular carcinoma and portal vein tumoral thrombosis: a pilot study. Liver Transplant 2021;27(12):1758–66.

33. Nordness MF, Hamel S, Godfrey CM, et al. Fatal hepatic necrosis after nivolumab as a bridge to liver transplant for HCC: are checkpoint inhibitors safe for the pre-transplant patient? Am J Transplant 2020;20(3):879–83.

34. Qiao ZY, Zhang ZJ, Lv ZC, et al. Neoadjuvant programmed cell death 1 (PD-1) inhibitor treatment in patients with hepatocellular carcinoma before liver transplant: a cohort study and literature review. Front Immunol 2021;12:653437.

35. Tabrizian P, Florman SS, Schwartz ME. PD-1 inhibitor as bridge therapy to liver transplantation? Am J Transplant 2021;21(5):1979–80.

36. Zhang XP, Gao YZ, Chen ZH, et al. An Eastern Hepatobiliary Surgery Hospital/portal vein tumor thrombus scoring system as an aid to decision making on hepatectomy for hepatocellular carcinoma patients with portal vein tumor thrombus: a multicenter study. Hepatology 2019;69(5):2076–90.

37. Lee KT, Lu YW, Wang SN, et al. The effect of preoperative transarterial chemoembolization of resectable hepatocellular carcinoma on clinical and economic outcomes. J Surg Oncol 2009;99(6):343–50.
38. Sasaki A, Iwashita Y, Shibata K, et al. Preoperative transcatheter arterial chemoembolization reduces long-term survival rate after hepatic resection for resectable hepatocellular carcinoma. Eur J Surg Oncol 2006;32(7):773–9.
39. Labgaa I, Tabrizian P, Titano J, et al. Feasibility and safety of liver transplantation or resection after transarterial radioembolization with Yttrium-90 for unresectable hepatocellular carcinoma. HPB (Oxford) 2019;21(11):1497–504.
40. Kaseb AO, Vence L, Blando J, et al. Immunologic correlates of pathologic complete response to preoperative immunotherapy in hepatocellular carcinoma. Cancer Immunol Res 2019;7(9):1390–5.
41. Kaseb AO, Cao HST, Mohamed YI, et al. Final results of a randomized, open label, perioperative phase II study evaluating nivolumab alone or nivolumab plus ipilimumab in patients with resectable HCC. J Clin Oncol 2020;38(15_suppl): 4599.
42. Pinato DJ, Fessas P, Sapisochin G, et al. Perspectives on the neoadjuvant use of immunotherapy in hepatocellular carcinoma. Hepatology 2021;74(1):483–90.
43. Li S, Zhong C, Li Q, et al. Neoadjuvant transarterial infusion chemotherapy with FOLFOX could improve outcomes of resectable BCLC stage A/B hepatocellular carcinoma patients beyond Milan criteria: an interim analysis of a multi-center, phase 3, randomized, controlled clinical trial. J Clin Oncol 2021;39(15_suppl): 4008.
44. Xu X-F, Xing H, Han J, et al. Risk factors, patterns, and outcomes of late recurrence after liver resection for hepatocellular carcinoma: a multicenter study from China. JAMA Surg 2019;154(3):209–17.
45. Han J, Fan YC, Wang K. Radiofrequency ablation versus microwave ablation for early stage hepatocellular carcinoma: a PRISMA-compliant systematic review and meta-analysis. Medicine (Baltimore) 2020;99(43):e22703.
46. Feng Y, Wang L, Lv H, et al. Microwave ablation versus radiofrequency ablation for perivascular hepatocellular carcinoma: a propensity score analysis. HPB (Oxford) 2021;23(4):512–9.
47. Livraghi T, Meloni F, Di Stasi M, et al. Sustained complete response and complications rates after radiofrequency ablation of very early hepatocellular carcinoma in cirrhosis: is resection still the treatment of choice? Hepatology 2008; 47(1):82–9.
48. Cho YK, Kim JK, Kim MY, et al. Systematic review of randomized trials for hepatocellular carcinoma treated with percutaneous ablation therapies. Hepatology 2009;49(2):453–9.
49. Shin SW, Ahn KS, Kim SW, et al. Liver resection versus local ablation therapies for hepatocellular carcinoma within the Milan criteria: a systematic review and meta-analysis. Ann Surg 2021;273(4):656–66.
50. Llovet JM, De Baere T, Kulik L, et al. Locoregional therapies in the era of molecular and immune treatments for hepatocellular carcinoma. Nat Rev Gastroenterol Hepatol 2021;18(5):293–313.
51. Wang C, Wang H, Yang W, et al. Multicenter randomized controlled trial of percutaneous cryoablation versus radiofrequency ablation in hepatocellular carcinoma. Hepatology 2015;61(5):1579–90.
52. Kim R, Kang TW, Cha DI, et al. Percutaneous cryoablation for perivascular hepatocellular carcinoma: therapeutic efficacy and vascular complications. Eur Radiol 2019;29(2):654–62.

53. Peng ZW, Zhang YJ, Chen MS, et al. Radiofrequency ablation with or without transcatheter arterial chemoembolization in the treatment of hepatocellular carcinoma: a prospective randomized trial. J Clin Oncol 2013;31(4):426–32.
54. Chen K, Chen G, Wang H, et al. Increased survival in hepatocellular carcinoma with iodine-125 implantation plus radiofrequency ablation: a prospective randomized controlled trial. J Hepatol 2014;61(6):1304–11.
55. Li Q, Chen K, Huang W, et al. Minimally invasive photothermal ablation assisted by laparoscopy as an effective preoperative neoadjuvant treatment for orthotopic hepatocellular carcinoma. Cancer Lett 2021;496:169–78.
56. Qi S, Zhang Y, Liu G, et al. Plasmonic-doped melanin-mimic for CXCR4-targeted NIR-II photoacoustic computed tomography-guided photothermal ablation of orthotopic hepatocellular carcinoma. Acta Biomater 2021;129:245–57.
57. Salem R, Johnson GE, Kim E, et al. Yttrium-90 radioembolization for the treatment of solitary, unresectable HCC: the LEGACY study. Hepatology 2021;74(5):2342–52.
58. Garin E, Tselikas L, Guiu B, et al. Personalised versus standard dosimetry approach of selective internal radiation therapy in patients with locally advanced hepatocellular carcinoma (DOSISPHERE-01): a randomised, multicentre, open-label phase 2 trial. Lancet Gastroenterol Hepatol 2021;6(1):17–29.
59. Dhondt E, Lambert B, Hermie L, et al. (90)Y radioembolization versus drug-eluting bead chemoembolization for unresectable hepatocellular carcinoma: results from the TRACE phase II randomized controlled trial. Radiology 2022;303(3):699–710.
60. Lee J, Shin IS, Yoon WS, et al. Comparisons between radiofrequency ablation and stereotactic body radiotherapy for liver malignancies: meta-analyses and a systematic review. Radiother Oncol 2020;145:63–70.
61. Yoon SM, Ryoo BY, Lee SJ, et al. Efficacy and safety of transarterial chemoembolization plus external beam radiotherapy vs sorafenib in hepatocellular carcinoma with macroscopic vascular invasion: a randomized clinical trial. JAMA Oncol 2018;4(5):661–9.
62. Soin AS, Bhangui P, Kataria T, et al. Experience with LDLT in patients with hepatocellular carcinoma and portal vein tumor thrombosis postdownstaging. Transplantation 2020;104(11):2334–45. https://doi.org/10.1097/tp.0000000000003162.
63. Kudo M, Ueshima K, Ikeda M, et al. TACTICS: final overall survival (OS) data from a randomized, open label, multicenter, phase II trial of transcatheter arterial chemoembolization (TACE) therapy in combination with sorafenib as compared with TACE alone in patients (pts) with hepatocellular carcinoma (HCC). J Clin Oncol 2021;39(3_suppl):270.
64. Peng Z, Fan W, Zhu B, et al. Lenvatinib combined with transarterial chemoembolization as first-line treatment of advanced hepatocellular carcinoma: a phase 3, multicenter, randomized controlled trial. J Clin Oncol 2022;40(4_suppl):380.
65. Finn RS, Ikeda M, Zhu AX, et al. Phase Ib study of lenvatinib plus pembrolizumab in patients with unresectable hepatocellular carcinoma. J Clin Oncol 2020;38(26):2960–70.
66. Lee I-C, Wu C-J, Chen S-C, et al. Lenvatinib plus pembrolizumab versus lenvatinib in patients with unresectable hepatocellular carcinoma: a real world study. J Clin Oncol 2021;39(15_suppl):e16138.
67. D'Alessio A, Fulgenzi CAM, Nishida N, et al. Preliminary evidence of safety and tolerability of atezolizumab plus bevacizumab in patients with hepatocellular carcinoma and Child-Pugh A and B cirrhosis: a real-world study. Hepatology. n/a(n/a)doi:https://doi.org/10.1002/hep.32468

Evaluation of an Abnormal Liver Panel After Liver Transplantation

Jacqueline B. Henson, MD[a], Andrew J. Muir, MD[a,b],*

KEYWORDS

- Liver transplantation • Liver tests • Primary nonfunction • Hepatic artery thrombosis
- Biliary complications • Recurrent disease

KEY POINTS

- The differential diagnosis and evaluation of an abnormal liver panel after liver transplant should be guided by the time course, pattern and degree of injury, and other aspects of the clinical picture.
- The initial diagnostic evaluation generally includes a liver ultrasound with Doppler to evaluate vascular patency, the hepatic parenchyma, and the biliary system, as well as additional laboratory testing appropriate to the clinical scenario.
- If the etiology is not determined after appropriate imaging and laboratory testing, a liver biopsy should be performed.

INTRODUCTION

Abnormal liver tests are common after liver transplantation, with many possible etiologies, including vascular issues, biliary complications, and causes of allograft parenchymal damage. The differential varies depending on the clinical context, particularly the time course, pattern and degree of elevation, donor and recipient factors, and other aspects of the clinical picture (**Fig. 1**). The perioperative period has distinct causes compared with weeks and years after the transplant. In this review, we explore the differential diagnosis for abnormal liver tests after a liver transplant and provide an approach to the diagnostic evaluation.

DIFFERENTIAL DIAGNOSIS
Perioperative period

The causes of abnormal liver tests in the immediate postoperative period are limited. In the days following transplant, ischemia-reperfusion injury is expected, though this

[a] Division of Gastroenterology, Department of Medicine, Duke University, DUMC Box 3913, Durham, NC 27710, USA; [b] Duke Clinical Research Institute, Duke University, DUMC Box 3913, Durham, NC 27710, USA
* Corresponding author. Duke University, DUMC Box 3913, Durham, NC 27710.
E-mail address: andrew.muir@duke.edu
Twitter: @jackie_henson (J.B.H.); @AMuir_DukeGI (A.J.M.)

Clin Liver Dis 27 (2023) 103–115
https://doi.org/10.1016/j.cld.2022.08.006
1089-3261/23/© 2022 Elsevier Inc. All rights reserved.

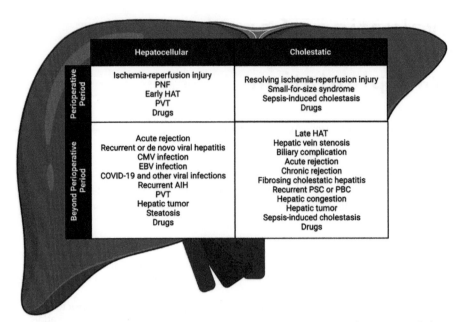

Fig. 1. Etiologies of abnormal liver tests in a liver transplant recipient by pattern of elevation and time course. COVID-19, coronavirus disease-2019.

should typically resolve within the first week. Failure to improve, other signs of graft failure, or improvement followed by worsening should prompt evaluation for other etiologies, including primary graft nonfunction (PNF) and vascular occlusion.

Ischemia-reperfusion injury

Liver allografts almost universally experience ischemia-reperfusion injury as a result of the organ procurement and transplantation process, with the degree of hepatocyte damage in proportion to the ischemic time. As a result, donation after cardiac death (DCD) grafts tends to have a greater injury than donation after brain death organs. Ischemia-reperfusion injury manifests as elevated transaminases (often >1000) in a hepatocellular pattern that typically peak after 1 to 2 days before rapidly declining and normalizing by 3 to 5 days after transplant, along with improving international normalized ratio (INR) and bilirubin. In some cases, there is prolonged cholestasis, though this will slowly improve more than 1 to 2 weeks if the injury is not severe.

Although ischemia-reperfusion injury typically improves, approximately 20% may experience early graft dysfunction, defined as either bilirubin ≥10 mg/dL on day 7, INR ≥1.6 on day 7, or aminotransferases greater than 2000 IU/L within the first 7 days.[1–4] The risk of early graft dysfunction increases with greater cold ischemic time, graft steatosis, and donor age, among other identified risk factors.[1–3] In many cases, ischemia-reperfusion injury and early graft dysfunction will not significantly impact long-term outcomes, but the severe injury is associated with inferior short-term graft survival and an increased risk of PNF.[1–3]

Primary graft nonfunction

Primary nonfunction is severe, irreversible early graft dysfunction that affects approximately 2% of recipients and is typically fatal without urgent retransplantation.[5] It manifests as markedly elevated transaminases in the several thousands and signs of liver failure with associated coagulopathy, encephalopathy, hypoglycemia, metabolic acidosis, and hemodynamic instability within the first week after transplant. For the purposes of status 1a designation, the Organ Procurement and Transplantation Network defines PNF as aspartate aminotransferase (AST) ≥3000 and either INR ≥2.5, arterial pH ≤7.30, venous pH ≤7.25, or lactate ≥4 within 7 days posttransplant. Diagnosis requires excluding other causes of graft injury, including hepatic artery thrombosis (HAT). Risk factors for PNF include donor age, donor illness severity, cold ischemic time, graft steatosis, as well as recipient illness severity.[5]

Early hepatic artery thrombosis

HAT can occur in the first 2 weeks after transplantation (early HAT) or in the later postoperative period (late HAT). Early HAT affects approximately 5% of recipients and causes severe graft dysfunction, with profound elevation in transaminases in a hepatocellular pattern due to ischemia.[6–8] The risk of HAT is increased by complex arterial anatomy, multiple arterial anastomoses, retransplantation, prolonged operation time, and in pediatric recipients.[6–8] Diagnosis can be made with a Doppler ultrasound and confirmed with computed tomography angiography (CTA) or magnetic resonance angiography (MRA). The prognosis is poor without urgent revascularization or retransplantation.

Portal vein thrombosis

Portal vein thrombosis (PVT) is less common than HAT, affecting 2% of transplant recipients.[7] As with HAT, it occurs most commonly in the early postoperative period but can also develop later. Approximately 60% with a PVT will have elevated transaminases, often mild or moderate though can be severe, whereas others present with complications of portal hypertension such as ascites or gastrointestinal bleeding.[7] Risk factors include small portal vein size, vascular redundancy, and preexisting PVT. PVT presents a technical challenge to retransplantation, though this may be required if other modalities such as thrombectomy or vascular reconstruction are unsuccessful.

Small-for-size syndrome

In the case of split/reduced grafts or living donor liver transplantation, small-for-size syndrome occurs when the functional mass of the graft is insufficient to support the needs of the recipient. This manifests as prolonged cholestasis (with bilirubin >5 for three consecutive days within the first week or at day 14) as well as other features of functional insufficiency such as ascites, coagulopathy, and encephalopathy.[9,10] The risk is increased with a graft weight to body weight ratio of less than 0.8, and the mechanism may be related to excessive portal inflow causing sinusoidal endothelial injury.[9,10] In some cases, the clinical features resolve as the graft regenerates, though the mortality rate is high.

Beyond the perioperative period

Vascular complications

Late hepatic artery thrombosis. In contrast to the rapid graft failure seen in early HAT, late HAT typically presents more indolently 1 to 12 months after transplant with biliary complications due to reliance of the bile ducts on the hepatic artery for blood supply. These complications range from asymptomatic cholestasis to symptomatic ischemic cholangiopathy, including jaundice, cholangitis, hepatic abscesses, sepsis, and biloma formation.[6] Diagnosis is made on Doppler ultrasound, CTA, or MRA. Liver retransplantation may be required in the event of hepatic failure or ischemic complications.

Hepatic vein/vena caval stenosis. Stenosis of the hepatic vein or inferior vena cava can occur when the surgery involves preservation of the recipient inferior vena cava ("piggyback technique"). The "piggyback syndrome" presents with signs and symptoms of venous outflow obstruction, including ascites, lower extremity edema, and predominantly mild-to-moderate cholestasis, usually in the first 3 months posttransplant.

Biliary complications

Biliary complications are common following liver transplant and affect an estimated 10% to 15% of deceased donor transplants and 15% to 30% of living donor recipients.[11] These include bile leaks, strictures, as well as biliary issues seen in non-transplant recipients such as choledocholithiasis. The bile ducts depend solely on arterial blood supply and therefore are particularly vulnerable to ischemic injury.[12] Biliary complications may manifest as asymptomatic cholestasis or be accompanied by jaundice, fever, pain, and sepsis.

Bile leaks. Most bile leaks develop in the first 1 to 3 months posttransplant and can occur at the anastomotic site (most common), cystic duct, or the cut surface of living donor grafts.[13] Anastomotic and cystic duct leaks are usually due to technical issues or ischemia. Bile leaks are typically symptomatic, with fever, pain, and jaundice. Biloma formation can cause biliary obstruction with associated mild-to-moderate cholestasis, depending on the size and location, and significant leaks can result in peritonitis.[11] The diagnosis is often made with a visualized fluid collection on ultrasound imaging, CT, or magnetic resonance cholangiopancreatography (MRCP), but hepatobiliary scintigraphy may be useful if these are equivocal.[12] Bile leaks are managed with endoscopic stent placement or percutaneous drain if endoscopic retrograde cholangiopancreatography (ERCP) is not feasible.

Biliary strictures. Biliary strictures can occur at the anastomotic site or elsewhere within the biliary tree (non-anastomotic strictures) and usually manifest within 2 to 6 months after transplant.[14] Anastomotic strictures may be the result of technical problems, ischemia, fibrosis, or prior bile leak, whereas non-anastomotic strictures are typically related to ischemia due to HAT (>50%), chronic rejection, or recurrent primary sclerosing cholangitis (PSC).[12] The risk of non-anastomotic strictures is also increased in DCD donors.[15,16]

Biliary strictures present with a mild-to-moderate cholestatic elevation in liver tests, which may be asymptomatic or with associated cholangitis. Diagnostic evaluation typically begins with a liver ultrasound with Doppler to also evaluate vascular patency, though bile ducts in the transplanted graft are less likely to be dilated in the setting of a biliary stricture. Ultrasound therefore has lower sensitivity to identify a stricture in transplanted grafts compared with native organs, so a normal study should be followed by MRCP and/or cholangiography if there is high clinical suspicion.[17] Treatment of anastomotic strictures involves balloon dilation and stent placement.[12] Management of non-anastomotic strictures depends on the location and extent of involvement but may involve endoscopic or percutaneous dilation/stent placement, antibiotic prophylaxis, and, ultimately, liver retransplantation.[12]

Rejection

Acute rejection. Acute T-cell-mediated rejection (TCMR) typically occurs beyond the first week postoperatively though within the first 90 days (early TCMR), but it can be seen up to 1-year posttransplant (late TCMR).[18,19] It affects 10% to 30% of recipients, with an increased risk in younger recipients and immune-mediated etiologies of liver disease and decreased risk in biologically-related living donor recipients.[18] The most common clinical presentation is asymptomatic elevated liver tests, though some may present with fever, malaise, and jaundice. The liver tests may be in any pattern, and the degree of elevation does not necessarily correlate with severity.[20,21] Imaging is typically performed to rule out vascular thrombosis or biliary stricture, but the diagnosis requires a liver biopsy. Histopathologic findings include portal inflammation, ductular inflammation, and endothelitis.[22]

Antibody-mediated rejection (AMR) is a rare cause of graft injury (<1%) in ABO blood group-compatible liver transplant that should be considered in patients with acute rejection not responding to standard therapy.[18] Diagnosis requires classic histologic features (endothelial cell hypertrophy/enlargement, capillary dilation, leukocyte sludging, and edema), complement four-dimensional vascular staining, circulating donor-specific antibodies, and exclusion of other causes.[19]

Chronic rejection. Chronic TCMR usually evolves from severe or persistent acute rejection and is observed in 1% to 5% of liver transplant recipients.[18] It involves potentially irreversible bile duct and/or vascular injury and manifests as progressive (initially mild) cholestasis, often in individuals with prior TCMR episodes and inadequate immunosuppression. Diagnosis is made on liver biopsy, and chronic rejection is characterized by ductopenia and perivenular inflammation and fibrosis.[19,23]

The diagnosis of chronic AMR is challenging as the histologic findings are not specific and may be present in recipients without rejection.[18,19] It should be suspected in recipients with persistent circulating donor-specific antibodies.

Recurrent disease

Recurrent disease should be considered as a cause of abnormal liver tests in the months to years following transplant. This is seen universally with untreated hepatitis C virus (HCV) infection and can also occur with hepatitis B virus (HBV) infection, PSC, primary biliary cholangitis (PBC), autoimmune hepatitis (AIH), nonalcoholic fatty liver disease (NAFLD), and alcohol-related liver disease, which generally present similarly as before transplant.

Hepatitis C infection. Before the development of direct-acting antiviral (DAA) therapies, recurrent HCV was the most common cause of graft loss and death in transplant recipients with HCV.[24] Recurrence is universal in recipients with HCV viremia at the time of transplant. The clinical course is variable, though, without treatment, most develop an acute flare in transaminases and a rise in HCV viral load 4 to 12 weeks postoperatively, reflecting acute HCV, followed by improvement and progression to chronic hepatitis.[25] In many cases, the transaminases will remain persistently or intermittently mildly elevated in a hepatocellular pattern, though 30% may have normal levels despite evidence of histologic damage. The progression of fibrosis is accelerated compared with non-transplant recipients, and 10% to 30% develop cirrhosis after a median 5 years.[25] A severe variant of recurrent HCV infection, fibrosing cholestatic hepatitis, is characterized by severe hyperbilirubinemia in the context of high levels of serum HCV RNA, typically within the first 2 years following transplant. Without treatment, there is rapidly progressive hepatic failure and graft loss.

Hepatitis B infection. Similar to HCV, recurrence of HBV following transplant was previously nearly universal and led to progressive disease with graft loss.[26] However, it is now rare with the use of antiviral therapies before transplant and continuation of these indefinitely posttransplant.[27] Risk factors for recurrence include pre-transplant HBV DNA level, hepatocellular carcinoma, and viral resistance.[28] Recurrence is heralded by the appearance of hepatitis B surface antigen, though an associated undetectable HBV DNA generally indicates adequate suppressive therapy.[29]

Primary biliary cholangitis. Recurrence of PBC occurs in approximately 20% of recipients at 5 years and 30% at 10 years and is associated with inferior graft and recipient survival.[30,31] As before transplant, recurrent PBC typically presents with a mild cholestatic elevation in liver tests and may be accompanied by nonspecific symptoms of fatigue and pruritus. The diagnosis is made by characteristic findings on liver biopsy in a recipient with persistently positive anti-mitochondrial antibodies and exclusion of other causes of cholestasis, including biliary obstruction and chronic rejection.[32] Younger recipient age and use of tacrolimus may increase the risk of recurrent PBC.[30,31] Treatment with ursodeoxycholic acid leads to biochemical response, though its impact on graft survival is uncertain.[33]

Primary sclerosing cholangitis. PSC recurs in 15% to 20% of transplant recipients.[34,35] Like PSC pre-transplant, the clinical course is variable but typically manifests with progressive mild-to-moderate cholestasis and biliary strictures. The diagnosis of recurrent PSC is made by characteristic cholangiographic and histologic findings and excluding other etiologies of diffuse, non-anastomotic biliary strictures such as HAT; it can be challenging to distinguish from chronic rejection.[36] Risk factors are poorly understood but may include recipient age, recurrent acute rejection, cytomegalovirus (CMV) infection, intact colon, cholangiocarcinoma, and prolonged steroid use.[34,37,38] Recurrent PSC may progress to require retransplantation.

Autoimmune hepatitis. Recurrent AIH occurs in 20% to 30% of recipients and manifests as elevated transaminases, elevated immunoglobulin G, presence of autoantibodies, compatible histopathologic findings, and response to steroids, though the diagnosis is difficult to distinguish from rejection.[39,40] The presentation is typically mild-to-moderate but can be more severe.[40–42] More severe inflammatory activity pre-transplant and higher transaminases and immunoglobulin G levels may increase the risk of recurrent AIH.[40,43] De novo AIH posttransplant has also been described, particularly in children and in recipients of female grafts or older donors.[39,40]

Nonalcoholic fatty liver disease. Recurrent NAFLD develops in a significant proportion of transplant recipients, with reported 5-year incidence rates ranging from 59% to 100%.[44] As before transplant, it typically presents with mildly elevated transaminases in a hepatocellular pattern. Most have histologically mild lesions but nonalcoholic steatohepatitis may occur in approximately 30% and advanced fibrosis in 5% to 10%.[44,45] De novo NAFLD is also common posttransplant, affecting 20% to 30% of recipients, though, in contrast to recurrent NAFLD, only a minority develop nonalcoholic steatohepatitis or advanced fibrosis.[45] These high rates of NAFLD posttransplant are likely related to a preexisting metabolic milieu pre-transplant which is exacerbated posttransplant by immunosuppressant medications, particularly steroids, leading to a high prevalence of the metabolic syndrome.[46]

Infection
Viral hepatitis. In addition to recurrent HCV and HBV, transplant recipients can also acquire these infections de novo posttransplant, including in some cases from their donor. De novo viral hepatitis should be considered in cases of an acute hepatitis with moderate to severe elevation in transaminases or with persistent mild transaminase elevation. Nearly all HCV- or HBV-infected organs are recognized pre-transplant and managed with antiviral treatment or prophylaxis. In rare cases, however, donor HBV or HCV infection can be occult, particularly in the context of recent donor injection drug use.[47–49]

Although HCV-positive organs used to be reserved for recipients with HCV, the advent of DAA therapy has facilitated their use in HCV-negative recipients as a means of expanding the donor pool. In non-HCV viremic recipients, diagnosis of acquired HCV is made by the presence of HCV RNA, usually detected within 3 to 7 days posttransplant.[50,51] The timing of initiating HCV treatment posttransplant has varied from within days to several weeks.[52,53] If treatment is more delayed, evidence of acute and then chronic HCV infection with elevated transaminases in a hepatocellular pattern typically develops.[51,52] Cases of fibrosing cholestatic hepatitis have been reported in recipients of HCV-positive kidney transplantation, so this should be considered in the event of severe hyperbilirubinemia.[54]

Recipients of HBV core antibody positive organs who are surface antigen negative and do not have natural immunity receive antiviral prophylaxis to prevent hepatitis B reactivation. Without prophylaxis, the risk of de novo HBV is 58% to 77% in unvaccinated recipients of these organs and 20% in vaccinated recipients, which is reduced to 11% and 2%, respectively, with antiviral prophylaxis.[55,56] De novo HBV is heralded by the appearance of HBV surface antigen or HBV DNA.

Another viral hepatitis with unique features posttransplant is hepatitis E virus (HEV), which typically causes an acute infection, but chronic HEV can develop in more than 60% of infected transplant recipients.[57,58] Chronic HEV presents as persistently mildly elevated transaminases in a hepatocellular pattern and a detectable HEV RNA and, if unrecognized, can progress to cirrhosis. Chronic HEV is treated with a reduction in immunosuppression and with ribavirin.

Cytomegalovirus. CMV is a common cause of abnormal liver tests after liver transplant, particularly in the first 3 months posttransplant. Recipients who have previously had CMV infection and are seropositive may experience reactivation with immunosuppression, and individuals who are seronegative are at increased risk of acquiring CMV, particularly if they receive a graft from a CMV-seropositive donor. These recipients typically receive prophylaxis to prevent infection.

CMV infection can be present in the absence of signs/symptoms or can manifest as CMV syndrome or CMV end-organ disease. CMV syndrome is characterized by fever, fatigue/malaise, leukopenia or neutropenia, thrombocytopenia, atypical lymphocytes, and mild-to-moderate elevation in transaminases in a hepatocellular pattern.[59] Outside of CMV syndrome, CMV hepatitis presents with abnormal transaminases and evidence of CMV in the absence of other etiologies. CMV is detected most commonly via quantification of CMV DNA in the serum, though it can be absent in the serum and still cause end-organ disease in some circumstances. In these cases or when evaluation for other etiologies is needed, histopathology remains the gold standard for diagnosis of end-organ CMV disease.[59]

Epstein–Barr Virus. Epstein–Barr Virus (EBV) infection is commonly acquired in childhood and 90% of adults are seropositive.[48] Posttransplant, EBV-seronegative recipients can acquire EBV, usually in the first year. This may be asymptomatic or manifest as a febrile mononucleosis syndrome with associated atypical lymphocytosis, lymphadenopathy, pharyngitis, hepatitis with mild-to-moderate transaminase elevation, meningitis, or pancreatitis. Primary EBV infection posttransplant vastly increases the risk of posttransplant lymphoproliferative disease (PTLD), which occurs due to uncontrolled proliferation and clonal transformation of EBV-infected B cells.[48] PTLD can also occur in EBV-seropositive recipients due to reactivation in the context of immunosuppression. It may present with nonspecific constitutional symptoms, a mononucleosis-like syndrome, and symptoms related to the organ(s) of involvement, which often includes the liver in liver transplant recipients.[60] Diagnosis is suspected with a more marked elevation in serum EBV viral load and confirmed on pathology.

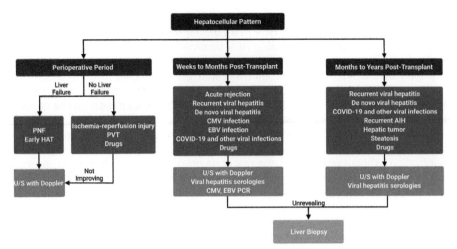

Fig. 2. Differential diagnosis and diagnostic evaluation of abnormal liver tests in a hepatocellular pattern in liver transplant recipients by time period. AIH, autoimmune hepatitis; COVID-19, coronavirus disease-2019; U/S, ultrasound.

Severe acute respiratory syndrome coronavirus 2 infection. Severe acute respiratory syndrome coronavirus 2 (SARS-CoV-2) infection can cause abnormal liver tests, usually a mild elevation in a hepatocellular pattern, and this is typically associated with more severe disease.[61] In liver transplant recipients, the degree and pattern of elevation is similar to non-transplant recipients, and these individuals are similarly likely to be hospitalized and to survive.[62,63]

Other infections. Transplant recipients are also at increased risk for other viral infections as well as bacterial and fungal infections, which can manifest with abnormal liver tests if there is hepatic involvement or a more systemic syndrome such as sepsis. These can be donor-derived, nosocomial, or community-acquired and should be considered according to the time period after transplant, the patient's epidemiologic exposures, and the degree of immunosuppression.[48]

Other etiologies
After transplant, recipients may also have abnormal liver tests from non-transplant-specific causes, including medications, alcohol, steatosis, hepatic congestion, and other etiologies.

DIAGNOSTIC EVALUATION

The diagnostic evaluation for abnormal liver tests posttransplant should be guided by the clinical scenario, including the time after transplant, the pattern and degree of elevation, donor and recipient factors, surgical technique, and other signs and symptoms. The first study obtained is generally a liver ultrasound with Doppler to evaluate vascular patency, the biliary tree, and the hepatic parenchyma. For a hepatocellular pattern of injury, viral hepatitis serologies should be obtained, including HBV (surface antibody, surface antigen, core antibody, as well as HBV DNA if known prior HBV or HBV core antibody-positive donor), HCV (anti-HCV antibody or HCV RNA if prior HCV infection, HCV-positive donor, or in the acute setting), as well as CMV and EBV DNA. If these tests are unrevealing, a liver biopsy should be obtained to evaluate for rejection or other etiologies. For a more cholestatic pattern of elevation, additional

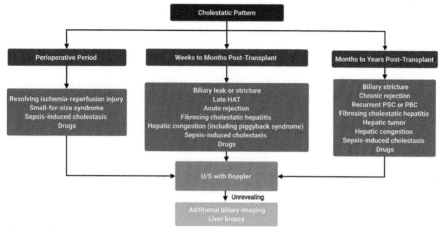

Fig. 3. Differential diagnosis and diagnostic evaluation of abnormal liver tests in a cholestatic pattern in liver transplant recipients by time period. U/S, ultrasound.

biliary imaging with MRCP may be useful, followed by ERCP if this is similarly inconclusive and for potential management. If the liver tests are only mildly elevated and the patient is otherwise well, this evaluation can occur in the outpatient setting.[64] If the injury is more severe or the patient has signs of liver dysfunction, however, inpatient evaluation is likely warranted. Diagnostic algorithms are shown in **Figs. 2** and **3**.

SUMMARY

In summary, there are many possible etiologies of abnormal liver tests after a liver transplant. The differential diagnosis and the evaluation should be guided by the time course, with unique causes in the immediate postoperative period, pattern of injury (hepatocellular vs cholestatic), and other aspects of the clinical picture. The initial diagnostic evaluation generally includes a liver ultrasound with Doppler to evaluate vascular patency, the hepatic parenchyma, and the biliary system, as well as additional laboratory testing appropriate to the clinical scenario. If the etiology remains uncertain after the appropriate imaging and laboratory testing, a liver biopsy should be performed.

CLINICS CARE POINTS

- Ischemia-reperfusion injury is expected, though this should typically resolve within the first week after transplantation.
- Primary nonfunction affects approximately 2% of recipients and is typically fatal without urgent retransplantation.
- Bile ducts in the transplanted graft are less likely to be dilated in the setting of a biliary stricture, and normal ultrasound should be followed by magnetic resonance cholangiopancreatography and/or cholangiography if there is high clinical suspicion.
- Antibody-mediated rejection is a rare cause of graft injury in ABO-compatible liver transplant that should be considered in patients with acute rejection not responding to standard therapy.
- In liver transplant recipients with severe acute respiratory syndrome coronavirus 2 infection, the degree and pattern of elevation is similar to non-transplant recipients

DISCLOSURE

JBH is supported by NIH grant 2T32DK007568-31A1.

REFERENCES

1. Ali JM, Davies SE, Brais RJ, et al. Analysis of ischemia/reperfusion injury in time-zero biopsies predicts liver allograft outcomes. Liver Transpl 2015;21(4):487–99.
2. Ito T, Naini BV, Markovic D, et al. Ischemia-reperfusion injury and its relationship with early allograft dysfunction in liver transplant patients. Am J Transplant 2021; 21(2):614–25.
3. Zhou J, Chen J, Wei Q, et al. The Role of ischemia/reperfusion injury in early hepatic allograft dysfunction. Liver Transpl 2020;26(8):1034–48.
4. Olthoff KM, Kulik L, Samstein B, et al. Validation of a current definition of early allograft dysfunction in liver transplant recipients and analysis of risk factors. Liver Transpl 2010;16(8):943–9.
5. Hartog H, Hann A, Perera MTPR. Primary nonfunction of the liver allograft. Transplantation 2022;106(1):117–28.
6. Mourad MM, Liossis C, Gunson BK, et al. Etiology and management of hepatic artery thrombosis after adult liver transplantation. Liver Transpl 2014;20(6): 713–23.
7. Duffy JP, Hong JC, Farmer DG, et al. Vascular complications of orthotopic liver transplantation: experience in more than 4,200 patients. J Am Coll Surg 2009; 208(5):896–903 [discussion: 903–5].
8. Bekker J, Ploem S, de Jong KP. Early hepatic artery thrombosis after liver transplantation: a systematic review of the incidence, outcome and risk factors. Am J Transplant 2009;9(4):746–57.
9. Hernandez-Alejandro R, Sharma H. Small-for-size syndrome in liver transplantation: new horizons to cover with a good launchpad. Liver Transpl 2016; 22(S1):33–6.
10. Hibi T, Kitagawa Y. Small-for-size syndrome in LT. Clin Liver Dis 2017;10(4):93–6.
11. Hampe T, Dogan A, Encke J, et al. Biliary complications after liver transplantation. Clin Transplant 2006;20(Suppl 17):93–6.
12. Seehofer D, Eurich D, Veltzke-Schlieker W, et al. Biliary complications after liver transplantation: old problems and new challenges. Am J Transplant 2013;13(2): 253–65.
13. Daniel K, Said A. Early Biliary complications after liver transplantation. Clin Liver Dis 2017;10(3):63–7.
14. Albert JG, Filmann N, Elsner J, et al. Long-term follow-up of endoscopic therapy for stenosis of the biliobiliary anastomosis associated with orthotopic liver transplantation. Liver Transpl 2013;19(6):586–93.
15. Detry O, Donckier V, Lucidi V, et al. Liver transplantation from donation after cardiac death donors: initial Belgian experience 2003-2007. Transpl Int 2010;23(6): 611–8.
16. Maheshwari A, Maley W, Li Z, et al. Biliary complications and outcomes of liver transplantation from donors after cardiac death. Liver Transpl 2007;13(12): 1645–53.
17. Potthoff A, Hahn A, Kubicka S, et al. Diagnostic value of ultrasound in detection of biliary tract complications after liver transplantation. Hepat Mon 2013;13(1): e6003.

18. Charlton M, Levitsky J, Aqel B, et al. International liver transplantation Society consensus Statement on immunosuppression in liver transplant recipients. Transplantation 2018;102(5):727–43.

19. Demetris AJ, Bellamy C, Hübscher SG, et al. 2016 Comprehensive Update of the Banff working Group on liver allograft pathology: Introduction of antibody-mediated rejection. Am J Transplant 2016;16(10):2816–35.

20. Abraham SC, Furth EE. Receiver operating characteristic analysis of serum chemical parameters as tests of liver transplant rejection and correlation with histology. Transplantation 1995;59(5):740–6.

21. Henley KS, Lucey MR, Appelman HD, et al. Biochemical and histopathological correlation in liver transplant: the first 180 days. Hepatology 1992;16(3):688–93.

22. Banff schema for grading liver allograft rejection: an international consensus document. Hepatology 1997;25(3):658–63.

23. Demetris A, Adams D, Bellamy C, et al. Update of the International Banff Schema for Liver Allograft Rejection: working recommendations for the histopathologic staging and reporting of chronic rejection. An International Panel. Hepatology. 2000;31(3):792–9.

24. Féray C, Caccamo L, Alexander GJ, et al. European collaborative study on factors influencing outcome after liver transplantation for hepatitis C. European Concerted Action on Viral Hepatitis (EUROHEP) Group. Gastroenterology 1999; 117(3):619–25.

25. Gane EJ. The natural history of recurrent hepatitis C and what influences this. Liver Transpl 2008;14(Suppl 2):S36–44.

26. Todo S, Demetris AJ, Van Thiel D, et al. Orthotopic liver transplantation for patients with hepatitis B virus-related liver disease. Hepatology 1991;13(4):619–26.

27. Young K, Liu B, Bhuket T, et al. Long-term trends in chronic hepatitis B virus infection associated liver transplantation outcomes in the United States. J Viral Hepat 2017;24(9):789–96.

28. Xu X, Tu Z, Wang B, et al. A novel model for evaluating the risk of hepatitis B recurrence after liver transplantation. Liver Int 2011;31(10):1477–84.

29. Fung J, Cheung C, Chan SC, et al. Entecavir monotherapy is effective in suppressing hepatitis B virus after liver transplantation. Gastroenterology 2011; 141(4):1212–9.

30. Corpechot C, Chazouillères O, Belnou P, et al. Long-term impact of preventive UDCA therapy after transplantation for primary biliary cholangitis. J Hepatol 2020;73(3):559–65.

31. Montano-Loza AJ, Hansen BE, Corpechot C, et al. Factors associated with recurrence of primary biliary cholangitis after liver transplantation and Effects on graft and patient survival. Gastroenterology 2019;156(1):96–107.e1.

32. Neuberger J. Recurrent primary biliary cirrhosis. Liver Transpl 2003;9(6):539–46.

33. Charatcharoenwitthaya P, Pimentel S, Talwalkar JA, et al. Long-term survival and impact of ursodeoxycholic acid treatment for recurrent primary biliary cirrhosis after liver transplantation. Liver Transpl 2007;13(9):1236–45.

34. Ravikumar R, Tsochatzis E, Jose S, et al. Risk factors for recurrent primary sclerosing cholangitis after liver transplantation. J Hepatol 2015;63(5):1139–46.

35. Hildebrand T, Pannicke N, Dechene A, et al. Biliary strictures and recurrence after liver transplantation for primary sclerosing cholangitis: a retrospective multicenter analysis. Liver Transpl 2016;22(1):42–52.

36. Graziadei IW, Wiesner RH, Batts KP, et al. Recurrence of primary sclerosing cholangitis following liver transplantation. Hepatology 1999;29(4):1050–6.

37. Liberal R, Zen Y, Mieli-Vergani G, et al. Liver transplantation and autoimmune liver diseases. Liver Transpl 2013;19(10):1065–77.

38. Steenstraten IC, Sebib Korkmaz K, Trivedi PJ, et al. Systematic review with meta-analysis: risk factors for recurrent primary sclerosing cholangitis after liver transplantation. Aliment Pharmacol Ther 2019;49(6):636–43.

39. Stirnimann G, Ebadi M, Czaja AJ, et al. Recurrent and de novo autoimmune hepatitis. Liver Transpl 2019;25(1):152–66.

40. Montano-Loza AJ, Ronca V, Ebadi M, et al. Risk factors and outcomes associated with recurrent autoimmune hepatitis following liver transplantation. J Hepatol 2022. https://doi.org/10.1016/j.jhep.2022.01.022.

41. Ratziu V, Samuel D, Sebagh M, et al. Long-term follow-up after liver transplantation for autoimmune hepatitis: evidence of recurrence of primary disease. J Hepatol 1999;30(1):131–41.

42. Hurtova M, Duclos-Vallée JC, Johanet C, et al. Successful tacrolimus therapy for a severe recurrence of type 1 autoimmune hepatitis in a liver graft recipient. Liver Transpl 2001;7(6):556–8.

43. Montano-Loza AJ, Mason AL, Ma M, et al. Risk factors for recurrence of autoimmune hepatitis after liver transplantation. Liver Transpl 2009;15(10):1254–61.

44. Saeed N, Glass L, Sharma P, et al. Incidence and risks for Nonalcoholic fatty liver disease and steatohepatitis post-liver transplant: systematic review and meta-analysis. Transplantation 2019;103(11):e345–54.

45. Pais R, Barritt AS 4th, Calmus Y, et al. NAFLD and liver transplantation: current burden and expected challenges. J Hepatol 2016;65(6):1245–57.

46. Azhie A, Sheth P, Hammad A, et al. Metabolic complications in liver transplant recipients: How we can Optimize long-term survival. Liver Transpl 2021. https://doi.org/10.1002/lt.26219.

47. Seem DL, Lee I, Umscheid CA, et al. PHS guideline for reducing human immunodeficiency virus, hepatitis B virus, and hepatitis C virus transmission through organ transplantation. Public Health Rep 2013;128(4):247–343.

48. Fishman JA. Infection in organ transplantation. Am J Transplant 2017;17(4):856–79.

49. Bixler D, Annambhotla P, Montgomery MP, et al. Unexpected hepatitis B virus infection after liver transplantation - United States, 2014-2019. MMWR Morb Mortal Wkly Rep 2021;70(27):961–6.

50. Kapila N, Menon KVN, Al-Khalloufi K, et al. Hepatitis C virus NAT-positive solid organ allografts transplanted into hepatitis C virus-negative recipients: a Real-World experience. Hepatology 2020;72(1):32–41.

51. Terrault NA, Burton J, Ghobrial M, et al. Prospective multicenter study of early antiviral therapy in liver and kidney transplant recipients of HCV-viremic donors. Hepatology 2021;73(6):2110–23.

52. Kwong AJ, Wall A, Melcher M, et al. Liver transplantation for hepatitis C virus (HCV) non-viremic recipients with HCV viremic donors. Am J Transplant 2019;19(5):1380–7.

53. Bethea E, Arvind A, Gustafson J, et al. Immediate administration of antiviral therapy after transplantation of hepatitis C-infected livers into uninfected recipients: Implications for therapeutic planning. Am J Transplant 2020;20(6):1619–28.

54. Kapila N, Al-Khalloufi K, Bejarano PA, et al. Fibrosing cholestatic hepatitis after kidney transplantation from HCV-viremic donors to HCV-negative recipients: a unique complication in the DAA era. Am J Transplant 2020;20(2):600–5.

55. Huprikar S, Danziger-Isakov L, Ahn J, et al. Solid organ transplantation from hepatitis B virus-positive donors: consensus guidelines for recipient management. Am J Transplant 2015;15(5):1162–72.

56. Skagen CL, Jou JH, Said A. Risk of de novo hepatitis in liver recipients from hepatitis-B core antibody-positive grafts - a systematic analysis. Clin Transplant 2011;25(3):E243–9.

57. Kamar N, Garrouste C, Haagsma EB, et al. Factors associated with chronic hepatitis in patients with hepatitis E virus infection who have received solid organ transplants. Gastroenterology 2011;140(5):1481–9.

58. Kamar N, Selves J, Mansuy JM, et al. Hepatitis E virus and chronic hepatitis in organ-transplant recipients. N Engl J Med 2008;358(8):811–7.

59. Razonable RR, Humar A. Cytomegalovirus in solid organ transplant recipients-guidelines of the American Society of transplantation infectious diseases community of Practice. Clin Transplant 2019;33(9):e13512.

60. Opelz G, Döhler B. Lymphomas after solid organ transplantation: a collaborative transplant study report. Am J Transplant 2004;4(2):222–30.

61. Bertolini A, van de Peppel IP, Bodewes FAJA, et al. Abnormal liver function tests in patients with COVID-19: Relevance and potential Pathogenesis. Hepatology 2020;72(5):1864–72.

62. Webb GJ, Marjot T, Cook JA, et al. Outcomes following SARS-CoV-2 infection in liver transplant recipients: an international registry study. Lancet Gastroenterol Hepatol 2020;5(11):1008–16.

63. Marjot T, Webb GJ, Barritt AS 4th, et al. COVID-19 and liver disease: mechanistic and clinical perspectives. Nat Rev Gastroenterol Hepatol 2021;18(5):348–64.

64. Graham DS, Busuttil RW, Kaldas FM. Outpatient management of liver function test Abnormalities in patients with a liver transplant. JAMA 2020;324(18):1896–7.

Noninvasive Fibrosis Testing in Chronic Liver Disease Including Caveats

Adam P. Buckholz, MD, MS, Robert S. Brown Jr, MD, MPH*

KEYWORDS

- Fibrosis • Elastography • Cirrhosis • HCC screening • Serum markers
- Test performance

KEY POINTS

- Fibrosis assessment is frequently important for determining risk and treatment strategy in those with chronic liver disease
- While imperfect, when used correctly non-invasive measures are generally appropriate to avoid a liver biopsy, which is itself an imperfect gold standard
- Appropriate understanding of test characteristics and patient circumstances can help apply the correct non-invasive fibrosis assessment tool

INTRODUCTION TO LIVER FIBROSIS ASSESSMENT

Given the persistence of cirrhosis as an important worldwide cause of morbidity and mortality, the accurate staging of liver disease is of paramount importance. Assessment of liver disease severity has improved significantly since the infancy of diagnosis in the mid-twentieth century with the discovery of alkaline phosphatase (ALP), alanine aminotransferase (ALT), and aspartate aminotransferase (AST) as well as initial use of liver biopsy. Now, a wide range of derived scores, laboratory examinations, and imaging options exist to help the clinician determine disease severity. This proliferation of diagnostic tools is of critical importance as the modern care of liver disease has evolved drastically. Our understanding of disease risk including decompensation and cancer, need for treatment, and even need for transplant rely on understanding liver disease state. Likewise, it's now widely accepted that hepatic fibrosis often exists in a dynamic state, with both progression or regression as potential outcomes at most time points in disease.[1,2] The sheer number of people with chronic liver disease, approximately 4.5 million Americans diagnosed excluding an estimated 30% of Americans with nonalcoholic fatty liver disease (NAFLD),[3,4] makes liver biopsy impractical for widespread assessment and monitoring of disease. This review will summarize

Division of Gastroenterology and Hepatology, NewYork-Presbyterian/Weill Cornell Medical Center, 1305 York Avenue 4th Floor, New York, NY 10021, USA
* Corresponding author.
E-mail address: rsb2005@med.cornell.edu

Clin Liver Dis 27 (2023) 117–131
https://doi.org/10.1016/j.cld.2022.08.008
1089-3261/23/© 2022 Elsevier Inc. All rights reserved.

the noninvasive methods for the evaluation of liver fibrosis. With numerous strengths and limitations of each diagnostic tool, clinicians treating chronic liver disease will use a vast array depending on circumstance, so this review will also discuss situations where usage of each may be ideal or inappropriate.

Situations Under Which Noninvasive Fibrosis Assessment is Used

This review will focus on fibrosis assessment for patient care rather than in evaluating eligibility and response in clinical trials, and the not-uncommon consultation for disease severity and risk evaluation in a patient with known chronic liver disease. In clinical care, fibrosis assessment is often performed on initial diagnosis and in follow-up for common diseases including alcohol-related liver disease (ARLD), viral hepatitis, NAFLD, primary sclerosing cholangitis, autoimmune hepatitis (AIH) and primary biliary cholangitis (PBC). It can also be helpful in the setting of liver disease diagnosed on imaging or laboratory assessment without a clear etiology. Similarly, fibrosis assessment may help to assess response to therapy in the case of hepatitis C or weight loss in the case of NAFLD. In addition, determining whether a patient has evidence of fibrosis can guide clinicians on whether to initiate therapy in the case of chronic hepatitis B (CHB) and whether to initiate hepatocellular carcinoma (HCC) screening in many liver diseases.

OVERVIEW OF TESTS OF LIVER FIBROSIS
Liver Biopsy as the Gold Standard

The accepted gold standard for assessment of hepatic fibrosis is histologic examination of a liver biopsy specimen. Such tissue is most often obtained either percutaneously, typically with ultrasound guidance, or transvenously, most often with passage of a transjugular catheter.[5] More recently, endoscopic ultrasound techniques have added an additional option for biopsy.[6] Regardless of tissue sampling method, liver biopsy has significant limitations in clinical use. Most notable is that it's invasive, with all techniques incurring an overall complication rate of 1% to 5%, including bleeding, pain or fever.[7] Likewise, there is significant expense and inconvenience incurred by the medical system and patient, respectively, even in the absence of complication. Also important, liver biopsy is a flawed gold standard. A recent study suggested that inter-rater reliability among pathologists for staging fibrosis was moderate at best, with a Cohen's kappa between 0.38 to 0.59.[8] This limits the ability of any noninvasive method to be studied conclusively against liver biopsy to determine its own reliability, and suggests that fibrosis has some subjectivity despite well-defined histopathologic criteria. In addition, there can be significant heterogeneity in fibrosis within a given liver, and the smaller the tissue sample, the more likely a biopsy will over or underestimate fibrosis. Therefore, all understanding of efficacy and utilization of surrogate tools must be couched in the realization that the reference standard is also imperfect. Despite this, liver biopsy remains the standard by which specific stages of fibrosis have been established including the widely accepted METAVIR score.[9] Use of a histologic standard with this score, which establishes standards for minimal fibrosis (F0 or F1), significant fibrosis (≥F2), advanced fibrosis (≥F3), and cirrhosis (F4), is also common in literature that has described the prognostic importance of various fibrosis stages across liver disease. Liver biopsy also remains the only test of fibrosis that also provides etiologic information as to cause of liver disease, so remains a critical diagnostic and prognostic tool. Because advanced fibrosis (≥F3) is known to be a major inflection point for clinical outcomes, including dictating initiation of HCC screening, noninvasive tests are often judged most critically on their ability to discriminate between advanced and non-advanced fibrosis.

Serum-Based Assessment of Fibrosis

The first serologic tests used to classify fibrosis were the AST and ALT in isolation and as a ratio, whereby a higher ratio of AST to ALT signified more significant and progressive liver disease.[10] However, it has now been well established that these liver enzymes are a marker of cell turnover and therefore have only indirect if any utility in detecting and staging fibrosis.[11] Likewise, decreased platelet count and elevated prothrombin time may indirectly suggest fibrosis and cirrhosis but have limited clinical utility in isolation.[12] Indirect markers of fibrosis may also be affected by other disease states, such as increase in bilirubin from Gilbert's syndrome.

In contrast, there are several serum tests that attempt to directly measure markers of hepatic fibrosis, thereby increasing detection capability and specificity. These include markers of matrix deposition such as procollagen I peptide, markers of matrix degradation such as matrix metalloproteinase-2 (MMP-2), and cytokines that stimulate fibrogenesis such as transforming growth factor alpha and beta. Such markers have been studied both in isolation and in combination. Although the full range of these tests is extensive and beyond the scope of this review, it should be noted that the accuracy of a blood-based marker can vary depending on the etiology of chronic liver disease. The FibroSpect test (a proprietary test including values for $\alpha 2$-macroglobulin, hyaluronic acid, and tissue inhibitor of matrix metalloproteinase-1), for example, uses different cutoffs for NAFLD than viral liver disease.

There are also several largely blood-based scores combining indirect or direct measurements of liver fibrosis with anthropomorphic data to provide a composite score. These include popularly used tests like the Fib-4 score (incorporating age) and NAFLD fibrosis score (age and body mass index (BMI)) as well as recently developed scores FibroMeter, which enhances predictive ability in NAFLD by including gender and weight along with commonly available blood tests like ferritin.

Imaging

By examining the appearance of the hepatic parenchyma using ultrasound, computed tomography or MRI, radiologists can provide morphologic interpretations that suggest fibrosis. In one study, volumetric measurement of liver and spleen for advanced fibrosis with computed tomography was relatively accurate.[13] Likewise, enhancement patterns on MR can be suggestive of fibrosis. However, these examinations have not been validated in the assessment of early fibrosis and can often be altered by concomitant diseases, inflammation, or motion.

Elastography

Elastography uses mechanical excitation of liver tissue in order to measure intrinsic stiffness as a function of resistance to the "shear wave" generated by the impulse. A multitude of techniques have been established, although the most common are vibration-controlled transient elastography (VCTE), marketed under the name FibroScan and MR elastography. VCTE uses a blunt tipped probe to emit a 50 mHz vibration shear wave and measures at a prespecified depth the velocity of the wave as it moves through the liver.[14] The velocity is then converted into a measure of liver stiffness in kilopascals (kPa) whereby a level of fibrosis can be inferred. MR elastography uses a driver device to pulse shear waves through the liver and then assess the pulsed wave using MR imaging. A quantitative algorithm is then used to interpret stiffness which correlates to different levels of fibrosis.

Two other important uses of elastography include acoustic radiation force impulse imaging (ARFI) and two-dimensional shear wave elastography (2D-SWE). ARFI uses a conventional ultrasound probe to deliver an acoustic pulse, with tissue displacement measured similarly to VCTE by the probe as an assessment of liver stiffness.[15] This allows it to be performed with a conventional ultrasound probe and can be therefore performed as a combined technique for image ascertainment. Another ultrasound-guided technique, 2D-SWE uses sequential geographically distinct ARFI measurements to build a two-dimensional image of the liver in real time while also examining a larger volume of tissue. This technique also uses conventional ultrasound probes and is therefore typically performed by experienced radiology departments.[16]

ADVANTAGES AND DISADVANTAGES OF ASSESSMENT OPTIONS

The three pillars of health care delivery are quality, cost, and access. All three vary by modality (**Fig. 1**) and may be considered in clinical decision-making for noninvasive assessment of fibrosis.

Quality

The quality of a noninvasive fibrosis assessment may be considered a combination of technical success rate, discrimination ability for fibrosis as measured by sensitivity and specificity, and the ability to precisely adjudicate stages of fibrosis. The indirect serum measurements of fibrosis tend to have high technical success rates but poor accuracy. For example, an AST/ALT greater than 1 has a sensitivity of 81.3% for identifying cirrhosis, but has a sensitivity of only 55.3% and cannot discern various stages of liver fibrosis.[17] Other blood-based markers, such as the AST-Platelet Ratio Index (APRI) tend to have better discriminative performance at higher levels of fibrosis. For example, in hepatitis C infected persons the discriminative ability for F2 fibrosis is much lower when measured as the area under receiver-operating curve (AUROC) than for cirrhosis (0.77 vs 0.83).[18] When these indirect markers are combined with other biometric data, the discriminative ability improves, often by including an "indeterminate" range. The NAFLD fibrosis score, for instance, uses a cutoff above 0.676 to suggest advanced fibrosis with a positive predictive value of 82% and a cutoff below −1.455 to suggest *no* advanced fibrosis with a negative predictive value of 88%.[19] Such accuracy may be helpful in avoiding a liver biopsy when in the "negative" range, but no such cutoffs have been established for early fibrosis. In addition, the test will fall

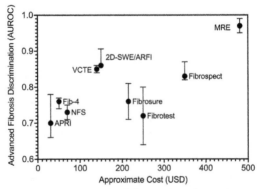

Fig. 1. Approximate cost and accuracy of noninvasive testing for advanced hepatic fibrosis. Although all areas under the curve (AUROC) with 95% confidence intervals are published in validation studies, there are several studies with different accuracies for each test. Likewise, the accuracy and cost of a specific test depend on the patient and disease, so these figures should be treated as approximations.

in the indeterminate range in 20% to 35% of recipients.[20] Among the most commonly used of the composite scores including indirect serum markers is the FIB-4 index, which combines ALT, AST, platelet count and age with a value >3.25 predictive of advanced fibrosis with a positive predictive value of 82.1% and a value <1.45 ruling out advanced fibrosis with a negative predictive value of 94.7%. The low "false negative" rate has made Fib-4 a popular initial screening test in chronic liver disease, although it should be noted that approximately 25% of tests will return an indeterminate value and 25% will be misclassified compared with a liver biopsy.

Many of the direct serum-based tests have improved performance relative to their indirect counterparts. In a prospective study comparing the FibroSpect II (with three direct markers of fibrosis) against the APRI with biopsy as a reference, FibroSpect II was far more accurate for identifying F2-F4 fibrosis (80.2% vs 48.4%), with a lower percentage of indeterminate results.[21] Again, however, most of these tests are developed to identify only advanced fibrosis, so although their accuracy is improved, they do not discriminate between stages and are more accurate in more advanced disease.

As above, most direct imaging modalities are unable to determine between stages of fibrosis. Alternatively, many of the elastography methods provide improved discriminatory ability along with the ability to ascertain specific fibrosis stages. At all stages, VCTE, ARFI, 2D-SWE and MRE tend to have an AUROC greater than 80%, and this accuracy tends to increase to approximately 90% at the stages of advanced fibrosis. Overall, the ultrasound elastography tests tend to have low level of discordance with liver biopsy for predicting fibrosis within two stages whether using ARFI or VCTE technology,[22] suggesting that the particular stage measurement has some clinical utility. It should be noted, however that it has been repeatedly showed that elastography techniques have high levels of reading overlap between contiguous stages of fibrosis.[23] MR elastography is felt to have the highest correlation with staging on histology, and has the possible advantage of not requiring "sampling" at a particular depth.[24] Unlike blood-based tests, imaging and elastography-based tests have a notable failure rate. VCTE has a reported failure rate of approximately 3%, often because of failure to find an adequate window for measurement or high variability in measurements. These failures are more common in more obese patients, and can be somewhat mitigated by usage of an XL probe which measures stiffness at a deeper point in tissue, obviating some issues of subcutaneous fat.[25] Failure rate is also higher with reduced operator experience and increased patient age. Ascites also increased failure rate but is seen more frequently in those with established cirrhosis.[26] MR elastography has a failure rate up to 5.5%, often in the case of technical failure, inadequate image resolution due to respiratory artifact or iron overload.[27] ARFI and 2D-SWE have reported failure rates of approximately 2%[28]; relative lower failure rates are believed to be because ascites can be accounted for, although failure rates may be higher in obese patients.[29] Excluding failures, MRE is felt to have the highest overall accuracy for detecting advanced fibrosis (AUROC >95%) and the highest accuracy for determining between stages of fibrosis of all noninvasive measures.[30]

Cost

There are a multitude of ways to measure cost of a test, including on the health system level, patient level, and as an effectiveness in reducing need for liver biopsy. These are beyond the scope of this review, which will focus on the billed cost of performing each test.[31] As a reference, cost of an image-guided liver biopsy, the standard of care, is approximately $1500.[32] From this perspective, indirect measurements tend to be the least costly, especially as they incorporate health care data routinely obtained in the management of chronic liver disease, such as weight, age, and liver enzymes.

Such testing often costs less than $100 per visit, with negligible additional cost for tests such as gamma-glutamyl transferase.[33] Costs for direct measurements of fibrosis are highly variable depending on the test, with many of the proprietary tests providing an interpretation of fibrosis costing significantly more than individual laboratory values. For example, FibroSure and Fibrospect II have reported average costs of $215 and $350, respectively.[34] Excluding equipment costs and focusing on billed costs, a VCTE (FibroScan) costs approximately $140, whereas MRE is $481.[35] The cost of ARFI and 2D-SWE likely approximates that of VCTE at approximately $150.[36] Several cost-effectiveness analyses have been performed in an attempt to incorporate test accuracy with cost in detecting advanced fibrosis and cirrhosis, with some suggesting initial evaluation with an indirect composite score such as the NAFLD fibrosis score or Fib-4 followed by VCTE or MRE for indeterminate or high values and biopsy reserved for any subsequent failures.[35] It should be noted, however, that as yet no clearly established cost strategy has incorporated all accepted testing modalities, and the least expensive testing choice may depend on patient characteristics and treatment setting.

Access

Choice of test when evaluating for fibrosis in chronic liver disease may be limited by test availability. Most practice settings whether inpatient or outpatient, academic or community, urban or rural will have access to basic laboratory and biometric testing in order to perform indirect tests of liver fibrosis including liver enzymes, GGT, age and weight. Thus, testing such as the APRI, Fib-4, and NAFLD fibrosis score are likely to be an attainable screening test even in the most resource-limited settings.[37] In addition, because many do not require a fasting state, serum evaluations may have improved immediate accessibility compared with elastography-based testing.[38] In stark contrast to the indirect markers, many if not all of the direct markers of fibrosis that have been validated in clinical practice are performed by private companies using a proprietary algorithm. Therefore, availability of testing and insurance coverage therein highly depend on the patient and setting. For example, in recently published clinical bulletin a major insurer (Aetna) describes some tests such as the FibroSure and enhanced liver fibrosis (ELF) score medically necessary, whereas others such as FibroSpect and HepaScore are considered investigational and not covered.[39]

For elastography-based methods, there is also significant variability in access based on setting. Because they use standard ultrasound probes, ARFI and 2D-SWE may be more readily available in inpatient settings compared with VCTE, but still requires specialized training and packaging on imaging systems, limiting utility in non-tertiary care settings. In recent years, several prominent manufacturers have begun integrating ARFI technology into their standard ultrasound which may improve access in the coming years, whereas Siemens now includes 2D-SWE on its clinical package.[40] MR elastography has several limits to accessibility including insurance approval, patient ability to receive an MR, and need for the specialized equipment to produce a shear wave.[41] One potential accessibility limitation for VCTE includes high upfront costs given the proprietary technology used (EchoSens, Paris, France), as well as variable insurance reimbursement for performance.[42] Alternatively, FibroScan requires less specialized training and is often available in real time to be performed at the bedside in less than 5 minutes.[43] There is no widely available data quantitating availability of testing methods by health care setting, so further research will be needed to better understand this spectrum of options. In the meantime, clinicians should consider the resources available at their own center when choosing a method for fibrosis assessment.

IMPORTANT CAVEATS WHEN CONSIDERING DIAGNOSTIC STRATEGY
Active Inflammation

In active inflammatory states such as nonalcoholic steatohepatitis (NASH), alcohol-induced hepatitis and chronic viral hepatitis, elevated ALT and AST may impact the accuracy of many testing modalities (**Fig. 2**). This is a significant contributor to the fact that ALT and AST cannot be used as valid screening tools, and active inflammation should make clinicians question the interpretation of tests such as Fib-4. Similarly, direct tests of fibrosis such as FibroTest may use values such as alpha-2-globulin (haptoglobin) which are altered in the setting of active inflammation and hemolysis, decreasing test accuracy.[44] Although elastography does not directly measure inflammatory markers, active inflammation may influence interpretation of shear wave promulgation. In one study evaluating VCTE in advanced fibrosis, an inflammation score greater than 2 on biopsy was associated with an odds ratio of 3.53 for misdiagnosis.[45] For this reason, ALT and AST values greater than twice the upper limit of normal may be unreliable in VCTE or require adjustment of thresholds, limiting clinical utility.[46] In one study, VCTE performed no better than Fib-4 or NAFLD Fibrosis score for identifying advanced fibrosis in those with ALT greater than 100. Fewer studies have evaluated the impact of inflammation on ultrasound-based techniques such as 2D-SWE, but these likely also have reduced accuracy in patients with elevated liver enzymes and/or known active inflammation and may require alternative thresholds to maintain accuracy for advanced fibrosis detection.[47] MR readings of elasticity can also be altered by presence of inflammation, such that accurate staging requires up to 3 to 6 months wait time after an acute inflammatory state.[48]

Disease State

Underlying etiology of liver disease is an important consideration in choice of test for fibrosis assessment. Many of the composite noninvasive markers of fibrosis have been validated only in a specific patient population. The Fibro Index, for one, was

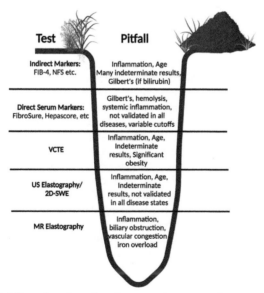

Test	Pitfall
Indirect Markers: FIB-4, NFS etc.	Inflammation, Age Many indeterminate results, Gilbert's (if bilirubin)
Direct Serum Markers: FibroSure, Hepascore, etc	Gilbert's, hemolysis, systemic inflammation, not validated in all diseases, variable cutoffs
VCTE	Inflammation, Age, Indeterminate results, Significant obesity
US Elastography/ 2D-SWE	Inflammation, Age, Indeterminate results, not validated in all disease states
MR Elastography	Inflammation, biliary obstruction, vascular congestion, iron overload

Fig. 2. Common pitfalls and confounders that provide a caveat for interpretation of several common noninvasive tests.

developed to identify advanced fibrosis in patients with hepatitis C, but had signifi-cantly reduced accuracy on validation and in a non-hepatitis C cohort.[49] Similarly, the APRI performed much more poorly among those with HCV if they were also co-infected with HIV.[18] If considering a serum biomarker, especially, it is important to consider whether the population in which published accuracies were established is applicable in the patient considered. A cutoff for every patient in every situation is probably impractical, which has served as a significant limitation for their implemen-tation in clinical decision-making. Similarly, Gilbert syndrome may falsely elevate serum tests that use bilirubin in their calculation of fibrosis.[50] Other systemic inflam-matory diseases may also increase some of the markers of fibrosis in the direct tests, such as urea and hyaluronate which are measured in Fibrometer and Hepascore, respectively.[51]

Separate cutoffs for advanced fibrosis are also used in VCTE, but have been well validated in PBC (>11 kPa),[52] NAFLD (>10 kPa),[53] PSC (>9.6 kPa), and hepatitis B/C/d (>9.5 kPa).[54,55] Preliminary data have suggested that VCTE may also be useful in fibrosis assessment in hemochromatosis, but further validation is needed.[56] Although further research is needed, VCTE is likely also valid for detecting advanced fibrosis in ARLD, but varying thresholds have been reported.[57,58] Caution should be taken in using elastography techniques in those with autoimmune liver diseases in the absence of clinical remission, as inflammation has been shown to alter stiffness measurements, but in treated AIH VCTE can likely be used for detecting advanced fibrosis (>10.5 kPa) and cirrhosis (>16 kPa).[59] Likewise, ARFI and 2D-SWE have been validated for use in both viral and nonviral chronic hepatitis for identifying advanced fibrosis.[60]

Several diseases are known to decrease elasticity readings (causing false elevations in assessment of fibrosis) with MRE. These include amyloidosis,[61] vascular conges-tion,[62] and biliary obstruction. For example, in patients with hyperbilirubinemia stiff-ness was on average 30% higher in one study, so consideration should be given to any obstructive physiology, especially in those with PSC.[63] Although MRE should be used with caution in patients with iron overload, a recent study suggests that use of spin-echo elastography sequencing can help to differentiate true fibrosis from iron overload.[64]

Patient Factors

Inherent patient factors may influence the accuracy of fibrosis assessments and there-fore choice of test. One important factor to consider is patient age, as most of the scoring cutoffs have been validated in those aged 35 to 65. It is known that some serum values including ALT and platelet count tend to decrease with age, regardless of liver disease. Inversely, these values are higher in younger patients, and one study has suggested that none of AST/ALT ratio, NAFLD Fibrosis Score, or Fib-4 were ac-curate in identifying advanced fibrosis in those younger than 35.[65] 'In the same study, NAFLD Fibrosis Score and Fib-4 showed rapid declines in specificity over age 65 as age is one of the calculated factors, decreasing clinical utility because of a high false positive rate. Older age was also noted to be significantly associated with decreased measurement reliability in US Elastography.[66]

Obesity, and BMI in general, can also complicate assessment of fibrosis. Increased waist circumference and abdominal fat increase the distance from the transducer probe to the liver ("skin to capsule") for elastography, especially VCTE and ARFI. In obese patients (BMI >30), VCTE has poorer discrimination and higher rates of false positives than in nonobese, with one recent study suggesting that use of the M versus XL probe did not mitigate this shortcoming.[67] MRE does not seem to have such shortcomings, with one study noting an accuracy of 95.8% for identifying advanced fibrosis in obese patients using MRE versus 81.3% in VCTE. They also noted that MRE performed better for differentiating stages of fibrosis than VCTE in those with morbid obesity.[68] Although data are mixed, it may be that US Elastography is more reliable in obesity than VCTE.[69] One study noted that elevated BMI did not decrease reliability but skin to capsule depth did, suggesting that the distance alone and no other patient factor was responsible for the unreliable measurement.[66]

Although presence of ascites may make readings of VCTE inaccurate, it is likely that those with ascites already are highly suspicious for a diagnosis of cirrhosis rather than fibrosis.[25] In the case of fibrosis assessment in a patient with ascites, MRE remains highly reliable. Finally, all elastography techniques should be performed fasting at least 3 to 4 hours given noted false elevations in elastography measurements post-prandially.[70] Likewise, direct tests of fibrosis that measure hyaluronate may be altered by recent intake, which can elevate serum levels.[71]

SUMMARY AND RECOMMENDATIONS

With recent advances in the treatment of chronic liver disease and the continued high prevalence and mortality of cirrhosis, fibrosis assessment has become increasingly important in clinical practice. Liver biopsy remains a valid tool, despite its shortcomings, expense, and risk profile. However, the ever-expanding toolkit of noninvasive options allows most patients to avoid a liver biopsy altogether. Unfortunately, the American Association for the Study of Liver Disease (AASLD) guidelines on use of liver biopsy predate many of the diagnostic and therapeutic advances of the last decade, and they do not have specific guidelines on fibrosis assessment. In 2015, the joint guidelines proposed by the European Association for the Study of the Liver (EASL) and Asociación Latinoamericana para el Estudio del Hígado (ASEH) acknowledge several situations where liver biopsy may be unavoidable, such as those when a measurement of portal pressure is needed, or when there are conflicting tests and liver biopsy is being used to clarify an uncertain result. At the time of publication of those guidelines, they posited that in diseases such as NAFLD the only clinically important endpoint was the presence or absence of cirrhosis. Since that time, the NASH Clinical Research Network has published a landmark study showing increased mortality even among those with F3 fibrosis.[72]

Such data highlights that the specific stage of fibrosis may be of interest in many circumstances, at which definition most of the serum biomarkers, especially the indirect markers, have high false positive and negative rates. Likewise, the frequency of indeterminate results makes scores such as the NAFLD fibrosis score difficult to use as a blanket tool. Despite this, several expert recommendations include use of an indirect serum biomarker as an initial "rule out" test for those at relatively low risk of advanced fibrosis, such as patients with NAFLD. In addition, serum biomarkers have been repeatedly shown to increase the performance of elastography tests when used in combination or in sequence.[73]

Therefore, the choice of first-line test will certainly depend on the specific patient situation as practice setting and resources and with consideration of the caveats for each test discussed above. For the average patient with known chronic liver disease, we have proposed a testing strategy for assessing advanced fibrosis (**Fig. 3**), given that this is often the most important prognostic marker for outcomes and to guide treatment. Among those in whom discrimination of a specific stage of fibrosis is desired (for example F1 or F2), there is no test that will provide absolute certainty. In fact, as mentioned above even the gold standard liver biopsy is fallible at such

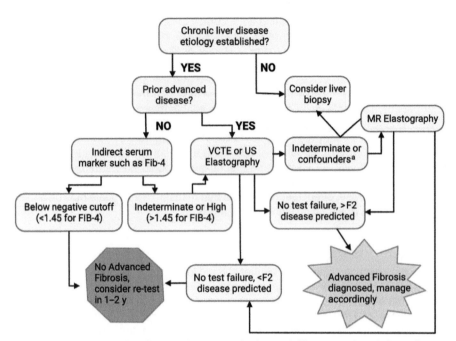

Fig. 3. Proposed algorithm for the diagnosis of advanced fibrosis in chronic liver disease. [a]Examples of confounders that may reduce accuracy of such methods are found in **Fig. 2.**

detail. Regardless, best evidence suggests that MR Elastography followed by ARFI and VCTE provides the best clarity on specific stage, whereas serum biomarkers are largely incapable of doing so. One important consideration in the algorithm proposed includes whether the patient has a known etiology of liver disease, because in the case of undiagnosed disease a liver biopsy may be cost-effective as a first step. Likewise, in a patient with previously known fibrosis or high risk for present fibrosis, such as a longstanding patient with hepatitis C undergoing assessment after sustained virologic response to treatment, serum biomarkers may be an inappropriate first step and progressing straight to elastography surveillance until fibrosis is felt to be minimal is recommended.

It is likely impossible to memorize all of the situations in which every biomarker has been validated or may be inadequate, as well as the various cutoffs that may signify fibrosis, indeterminate range, or no fibrosis. For this reason, it's more practical to become comfortable with the indications and usage of one or several of these tests, as research suggests that all are similarly adequate for ruling out advanced fibrosis when used appropriately. Considering cost, ease of use, and validation in multiple disease states, the Fib-4 index is likely appropriate first-line test in most circumstances. In all cases, it's important to properly communicate to patients that despite our overall improvement in assessing fibrosis noninvasively, test failure and incorrect or conflicting categorization can occur, making liver biopsy a valuable backup.

CLINICS CARE POINTS

- Liver biopsy samples only a limited portion of tissue, making it prone to error especially in patchy fibrosis/inflammation

- While non-invasive measures can sometimes help with diagnosis of liver disease etiology, circumstances with significant equipoise may call for a biopsy with additional fibrosis assessment
- Active inflammation (judged most frequently by elevated ALT and AST) may alter test performance for non-invasive assessments
- It is critical to consider whether the test of choice has been assessed and norms have been established for the particular disease state for which fibrosis assessment is desired

DISCLOSURE

The authors have nothing to disclose.

REFERENCES

1. Ellis EL, Mann DA. Clinical evidence for the regression of liver fibrosis. J Hepatol 2012;56(5):1171–80.
2. Tada T, Kumada T, Toyoda H, et al. Improvement of liver stiffness in patients with hepatitis C virus infection who received direct-acting antiviral therapy and achieved sustained virological response. J Gastroenterol Hepatol 2017;32(12):1982–8.
3. Younossi ZM, Stepanova M, Younossi Y, et al. Epidemiology of chronic liver diseases in the USA in the past three decades. Gut 2020;69(3):564–8.
4. Center for Health Statistics N, Table A-4. Selected diseases and conditions among adults aged 18 and over, by selected characteristics: United States, 2018. 2018. Available at: http://www.cdc.gov/nchs/nhis/SHS/tables.htm. Accessed April 23, 2022.
5. Rockey DC, Caldwell SH, Goodman ZD, et al. Liver biopsy. Hepatology 2009. https://doi.org/10.1002/hep.22742.
6. Shah AR, Al-Hanayneh M, Chowdhry M, et al. Endoscopic ultrasound guided liver biopsy for parenchymal liver disease. World J Hepatol 2019;11(4):335.
7. Boyum JH, Atwell TD, Schmit GD, et al. Incidence and risk factors for adverse events related to image-guided liver biopsy. Mayo Clin Proc 2016;91(3):329–35.
8. Davison BA, Harrison SA, Cotter G, et al. Suboptimal reliability of liver biopsy evaluation has implications for randomized clinical trials. J Hepatol 2020;73(6):1322–32.
9. Bedossa P. Intraobserver and Interobserver Variations in liver biopsy interpretation in patients with chronic hepatitis C. Hepatology 1994;20(1):15–20.
10. de Ritis F, Coltorti M, Giusti G. An enzymic test for the diagnosis of viral hepatitis; the transaminase serum activities. Clin Chim Acta 1957;2(1):70–4.
11. Reedy DW, Loo AT, Levine RA. AST/ALT ratio > or = 1 is not diagnostic of cirrhosis in patients with chronic hepatitis C. Dig Dis Sci 1998;43(9):2156–9.
12. Parkes J, Guha IN, Roderick P, et al. Performance of serum marker panels for liver fibrosis in chronic hepatitis C. J Hepatol 2006;44(3):462–74.
13. Pickhardt PJ, Malecki K, Hunt OF, et al. Hepatosplenic volumetric assessment at MDCT for staging liver fibrosis. Eur Radiol 2017;27(7):3060–8.
14. Afdhal NH. Fibroscan (transient elastography) for the measurement of liver fibrosis. Gastroenterol Hepatol 2012;8(9):605. Available at: http://pmc/articles/PMC3594956/. Accessed April 14, 2022.
15. Friedrich-Rust M, Wunder K, Kriener S, et al. Liver fibrosis in viral hepatitis: noninvasive assessment with acoustic radiation force impulse imaging versus transient elastography. Radiology 2009;252(2):595–604.

16. Gao Y, Zheng J, Liang P, et al. Liver fibrosis with two-dimensional US shear-wave elastography in participants with chronic hepatitis B: a prospective multicenter study. Radiology 2018;289(2):407–15.
17. Giannini E, Risso D, Botta F, et al. Validity and clinical utility of the aspartate aminotransferase–alanine aminotransferase ratio in assessing disease severity and prognosis in patients with hepatitis C virus–related chronic liver disease. Arch Intern Med 2003;163(2):218–24.
18. Lin ZH, Xin YN, Dong QJ, et al. Performance of the aspartate aminotransferase-to-platelet ratio index for the staging of hepatitis C-related fibrosis: an updated meta-analysis. Hepatology 2011;53(3):726–36.
19. Angulo P, Hui JM, Marchesini G, et al. The NAFLD fibrosis score: a noninvasive system that identifies liver fibrosis in patients with NAFLD. Hepatology 2007; 45(4):846–54.
20. Loomba R, Adams LA. Recent advances in clinical practice Advances in noninvasive assessment of hepatic fibrosis. Gut 2020;69:1343–52.
21. Patel K, Nelson DR, Rockey DC, et al. Correlation of FIBROSpect II with histologic and morphometric evaluation of liver fibrosis in chronic hepatitis C. Clin Gastroenterol Hepatol 2008;6(2):242–7.
22. Cassinotto C, Lapuyade B, Mouries A, et al. Noninvasive assessment of liver fibrosis with impulse elastography: comparison of supersonic shear imaging with ARFI and FibroScan Ò. Available at: www.biopredictive.com. Accessed April 17, 2022.
23. Zhang YN, Fowler KJ, Ozturk A, et al. Liver fibrosis imaging: a clinical review of ultrasound and magnetic resonance elastography. J Magn Reson Imaging 2020; 51(1):25.
24. Barr RG, Ferraioli G, Palmeri ML, et al. Elastography assessment of liver fibrosis: society of radiologists in ultrasound consensus conference statement. Radiology 2015;276(3):845–61.
25. Castéra L, Foucher J, Bernard PH, et al. Pitfalls of liver stiffness measurement: a 5-year prospective study of 13,369 examinations. Hepatology 2010;51(3): 828–35.
26. Afdhal NH. Fibroscan (transient elastography) for the measurement of liver fibrosis. Gastroenterol Hepatol 2012;8(9):605. Available at: http://pmc/articles/PMC3594956/. Accessed April 18, 2022.
27. Yin M, Glaser KJ, Talwalkar JA, et al. Hepatic MR elastography: clinical performance in a series of 1377 consecutive examinations1. Radiology 2016;278(1): 114–24.
28. Cassinotto C, Lapuyade B, Aït-Ali A, et al. Liver fibrosis: noninvasive assessment with acoustic radiation force impulse elastography–comparison with FibroScan M and XL probes and FibroTest in patients with chronic liver disease. Radiology 2013;269(1):283–92.
29. Ferraioli G, Tinelli C, Lissandrin R, et al. Ultrasound point shear wave elastography assessment of liver and spleen stiffness: effect of training on repeatability of measurements. Eur Radiol 2014;24(6):1283–9.
30. Xiao H, Shi M, Xie Y, et al. Comparison of diagnostic accuracy of magnetic resonance elastography and Fibroscan for detecting liver fibrosis in chronic hepatitis B patients: a systematic review and meta-analysis. PLOS ONE 2017;12(11): e0186660.
31. HERC: measuring costs for cost-effectiveness analysis. Available at: https://www.herc.research.va.gov/include/page.asp?id=measure-costs-cea. Accessed April 18, 2022.

32. Increasing Use of percutaneous liver biopsy accompanied by growing costs. Available at: https://www.hmpgloballearningnetwork.com/site/jcp/article/increasing-use-percutaneous-liver-biopsy-accompanied-growing-costs. Accessed April 18, 2022.

33. Tapper EB, Saini SD, Sengupta N. Extensive testing or focused testing of patients with elevated liver enzymes. J Hepatol 2017;66(2):313–9.

34. Carlson JJ, Kowdley Kv, Sullivan SD, et al. An evaluation of the potential cost-effectiveness of noninvasive testing strategies in the diagnosis of significant liver fibrosis. J Gastroenterol Hepatol 2009;24(5):786.

35. Vilar-Gomez E, Lou Z, Kong N, et al. Cost effectiveness of different strategies for detecting cirrhosis in patients with Nonalcoholic fatty liver disease based on United States health care system. Clin Gastroenterol Hepatol 2020. https://doi.org/10.1016/j.cgh.2020.04.017.

36. Congly SE, Shaheen AA, Swain MG. Modelling the cost effectiveness of non-alcoholic fatty liver disease risk stratification strategies in the community setting. PLOS ONE 2021;16(5):e0251741.

37. Salkic NN, Cickusic E, Jovanovic P, et al. Online combination algorithm for noninvasive assessment of chronic hepatitis B related liver fibrosis and cirrhosis in resource-limited settings. Eur J Intern Med 2015. https://doi.org/10.1016/j.ejim.2015.07.005.

38. Patel K, Sebastiani G. Limitations of noninvasive tests for assessment of liver fibrosis. JHEP Rep 2020;2(2):100067.

39. Noninvasive tests for hepatic fibrosis - medical clinical policy bulletins | aetna. Available at: http://www.aetna.com/cpb/medical/data/600_699/0690.html. Accessed April 18, 2022.

40. Nowotny F, Schmidberger J, Schlingeloff P, et al. Comparison of point and two-dimensional shear wave elastography of the spleen in healthy subjects. World J Radiol 2021;13(5):137.

41. Kennedy P, Wagner M, Castéra L, et al. Quantitative elastography methods in liver disease: Current evidence and Future Directions. Radiology 2018;286(3):738.

42. Return on Investment (ROI) of vibration-controlled transient... : Official journal of the American College of Gastroenterology | ACG. Available at: https://journals.lww.com/ajg/Fulltext/2017/10001/Return_on_Investment__ROI__of_Vibration_Controlled.950.aspx. Accessed April 18, 2022.

43. Pinzani M, Vizzutti F, Arena U, et al. Technology Insight: noninvasive assessment of liver fibrosis by biochemical scores and elastography. Nat Clin Pract Gastroenterol Hepatol 2008;5(2):95–106.

44. Poynard T, Morra R, Halfon P, et al. Meta-analyses of FibroTest diagnostic value in chronic liver disease. BMC Gastroenterol 2007;7:40.

45. Huang LL, Lin HM, Kang NL, et al. Effect of liver inflammation on accuracy of FibroScan device in assessing liver fibrosis stage in patients with chronic hepatitis B virus infection. World J Gastroenterol 2021;27(7):641.

46. Arena U, Vizzutti F, Corti G, et al. Acute viral hepatitis increases liver stiffness values measured by transient elastography. Hepatology 2008;47(2):380–4.

47. Zeng J, Zheng J, Jin JY, et al. Shear wave elastography for liver fibrosis in chronic hepatitis B: adapting the cut-offs to alanine aminotransferase levels improves accuracy. Eur Radiol 2019;29(2):857–65.

48. Venkatesh SK, Wells ML, Miller FH, et al. Magnetic resonance elastography: beyond liver fibrosis—a case-based pictorial review. Abdom Radiol (Ny) 2018;43(7):1590.

49. Imbert-Bismut F, Ratziu V, Pieroni L, et al. Biochemical markers of liver fibrosis in patients with hepatitis C virus infection: a prospective study. Lancet 2001; 357(9262):1069–75.
50. Rockey DC, Bissell DM. Noninvasive measures of liver fibrosis. Hepatology 2006; 43(S1):S113–20.
51. Volpi N, Schiller J, Stern R, et al. Role, metabolism, chemical modifications and applications of hyaluronan. Curr Med Chem 2009;16(14):1718–45.
52. Cristoferi L, Calvaruso V, Overi D, et al. Accuracy of transient elastography in assessing fibrosis at diagnosis in Naïve patients with primary biliary cholangitis: a dual cut-Off approach. Hepatology 2021;74(3):1496–508.
53. Tapper EB, Challies T, Nasser I, et al. The performance of vibration controlled transient elastography in a US cohort of patients with non-alcoholic fatty liver disease. Am J Gastroenterol 2016;111(5):677.
54. Evaluation de la. stéatose à partir du FibroScan® par un index ultrasonore de stéatose-validation sur une cohorte de 618 patients VHC. https://onlinelibrary. wiley.com/doi/full/10.1111/j.1365-2893.2011.01534.x.
55. Castéra L, Vergniol J, Foucher J, et al. Prospective comparison of transient elastography, Fibrotest, APRI, and liver biopsy for the assessment of fibrosis in chronic hepatitis C. Gastroenterology 2005;128(2):343–50.
56. Adhoute X, Foucher J, Laharie D, et al. Diagnosis of liver fibrosis using FibroScan and other noninvasive methods in patients with hemochromatosis: a prospective study. Gastroentérol Clin Biol 2008;32(2):180–7.
57. Mueller S, Millonig G, Sarovska L, et al. Increased liver stiffness in alcoholic liver disease: differentiating fibrosis from steatohepatitis. World J Gastroenterol 2010; 16(8):966.
58. Pavlov CS, Casazza G, Nikolova D, et al. Transient elastography for diagnosis of stages of hepatic fibrosis and cirrhosis in people with alcoholic liver disease. Cochrane Database Syst Rev 2015;1(1). https://doi.org/10.1002/14651858. CD010542.PUB2.
59. Hartl J, Denzer U, Ehlken H, et al. Transient elastography in autoimmune hepatitis: Timing determines the impact of inflammation and fibrosis.
60. Lin Y, Li H, Jin C, et al. The diagnostic accuracy of liver fibrosis in non-viral liver diseases using acoustic radiation force impulse elastography: a systematic review and meta-analysis. PLoS ONE 2020;15(1). https://doi.org/10.1371/ JOURNAL.PONE.0227358.
61. Peker E, Erden A. T1 mapping and magnetic resonance elastography: potential new techniques for quantification of parenchymal changes in hepatic amyloidosis. Diagn Interv Radiol 2017;23(6):478.
62. Babu AS, Wells ML, Teytelboym OM, et al. Elastography in chronic liver disease: modalities, techniques, limitations, and Future Directions. Radiographics 2016; 36(7):1987.
63. Kim DK, Choi JY, Park MS, et al. Clinical Feasibility of MR elastography in patients with biliary obstruction. AJR Am J Roentgenol 2018;210(6):1273–8.
64. Mariappan YK, Dzyubak B, Glaser KJ, et al. Application of modifed spinecho-based sequences for hepatic MR elastography: evaluation, comparison with the conventional gradient-echo sequence, and preliminary clinical experience. Radiology 2017;282(2):390–8.
65. McPherson S, Hardy T, Dufour JF, et al. Age as a confounding factor for the accurate noninvasive diagnosis of advanced NAFLD fibrosis. Am J Gastroenterol 2017;112(5):740.

66. Byenfeldt M, Elvin A, Fransson P. On patient related factors and their impact on ultrasound-based shear wave elastography of the liver. Ultrasound Med Biol 2018;44(8):1606–15.

67. Petta S, Wai-Sun Wong V, Bugianesi E, et al. Impact of obesity and alanine amino-transferase levels on the diagnostic accuracy for advanced liver fibrosis of nonin-vasive tools in patients with Nonalcoholic fatty liver disease. Am J Gastroenterol 2019;114(6):916–28.

68. Chen J, Yin M, Talwalkar JA, et al. Diagnostic performance of MR elastography and vibration-controlled transient elastography in the detection of hepatic fibrosis in patients with severe to morbid obesity. Radiology 2017;283(2):418.

69. Palmeri ML, Wang MH, Dahl JJ, et al. Quantifying hepatic shear modulus in vivo using acoustic radiation force. Ultrasound Med Biol 2008;34(4):546–58.

70. Obrzut M, Atamaniuk V, Chen J, et al. Postprandial hepatic stiffness changes on magnetic resonance elastography in healthy volunteers. Scientific Rep 2021; 11(1):1–7.

71. Fraser JRE, Gibson PR. Mechanisms by which food intake elevates circulating levels of hyaluronan in humans. J Intern Med 2005;258(5):460–6.

72. Sanyal AJ, van Natta ML, Clark J, et al. Prospective study of outcomes in adults with Nonalcoholic fatty liver disease. N Engl J Med 2021;385(17):1559–69.

73. Mózes FE, Lee JA, Selvaraj EA, et al. Diagnostic accuracy of noninvasive tests for advanced fibrosis in patients with NAFLD: an individual patient data meta-anal-ysis. Gut 2022;71(5):1006–19.

Evaluation of Liver Disease in Pregnancy

Gres Karim, MD[a], Dewan Giri, MBBS[a], Tatyana Kushner, MD, MSCE[b,c,*],
Nancy Reau, MD[d]

KEYWORDS

- Pregnancy • Preeclampsia • Nonalcoholic fatty liver disease • HELLP
- Hyperemesis gravidarum • Intrahepatic cholestasis of pregnancy

KEY POINTS

- The diagnostic approach to abnormal liver tests in pregnancy involves an assessment of liver injury pattern and evaluation for liver diseases unique to pregnancy.
- Liver diseases unique to pregnancy generally occur in specific pregnancy trimesters, but there are exceptions in timing of onset.
- Diagnostic criteria such as Swansea criteria for acute fatty liver disease of pregnancy and the Mississippi classification for HELLP can be helpful in the diagnostic workup of patients.
- There are specific management considerations for chronic liver disease both during pregnancy and in regards to breastfeeding in order to optimize disease and pregnancy outcomes.
- Portal hypertension in pregnant individuals can be associated with risk of variceal bleed in pregnancy; endoscopic evaluation should occur during pregnancy particularly if there is no endoscopy within a year prior to pregnancy.

Liver disease occurs in 5% to 10% of pregnancies and requires diagnostic and therapeutic considerations that may be unique to pregnancy. Liver injury in pregnancy can be broadly categorized into chronic liver disease, liver disease unique to pregnancy, and liver disease coincidental to pregnancy. Guidelines from both the American College of Gastroenterology[1] and the American Association for the Study of Liver Diseases (AASLD)[2] delineate diagnostic pathways and provide therapeutic recommendations for liver disease in pregnancy. There is ongoing clinical investigation to improve our understanding of the optimal strategies to address liver disease in

[a] Department of Medicine, Mount Sinai Beth Israel, 350 East 17th Street, 20th Floor, New York, NY 10003, USA; [b] Division of Liver Diseases, Icahn School of Medicine at Mount Sinai, One Gustave L Levy Place, Box 1123, New York, NY 10023, USA; [c] Department of Obstetrics, Gynecology, and Reproductive Sciences, Icahn School of Medicine at Mount Sinai, One Gustave L Levy Place, Box 1123, New York, NY 10023, USA; [d] Division of Hepatology, Rush University Medical Center, 1725 West Harrison Street | Suite 319, Chicago, IL 60612, USA
* Corresponding author. One Gustave L Levy Place, Box 1123, New York, NY 10023.
E-mail address: Tatyana.kushner@mssm.edu

Clin Liver Dis 27 (2023) 133–155
https://doi.org/10.1016/j.cld.2022.08.009
1089-3261/23/© 2022 Elsevier Inc. All rights reserved.

liver.theclinics.com

pregnancy and to optimize maternal and fetal outcomes. This review addresses our current knowledge of the evaluation of liver disease in pregnancy.

DIAGNOSTIC APPROACH TO LIVER DISEASE IN PREGNANCY

Evaluation of a pregnant woman without known liver disease will be similar to that of a nonpregnant individual although testing needs to balance risk to the mother and fetus against the information obtained and must be interpreted in the context of gestational age. Initial evaluation starts with a history (including medications and supplements), physical examination, and laboratory assessment. The history should assess for any known personal and family history of prior liver disease, risk factors for liver disease (such as injection drug use or other bloodborne exposures for hepatitis C or hepatitis B, metabolic risk factors for nonalcoholic fatty liver disease [NAFLD]), prior pregnancy history (such as prior history of complications of pregnancy such as preeclampsia), and/or symptoms during current pregnancy (ie, nausea, emesis, pruritus). Physical examination should focus on evaluating for any evidence of chronic liver disease such as scleral icterus or jaundice, advanced liver disease such as palmar erythema, ascites, or lower extremity edema, although this can be confounded by normal physical changes of pregnancy. The pattern of liver tests elevation, hepatocellular or cholestatic, then guides further testing (**Fig. 1**). When evaluating the prevalence of liver disease subtypes among cohorts of patients, the most prevalent cause of abnormal liver chemistries is actually gallstones and biliary disease followed by liver disease unique to pregnancy.[3–5] In addition, providers should be mindful that NAFLD is the most prevalent chronic liver condition among women of reproductive age, and therefore should be considered early in evaluation. Liver diseases unique to pregnancy will increase in prevalence in the second and third trimester and must be high on the differential.

LIVER DISEASES UNIQUE TO PREGNANCY

Liver disease unique to pregnancy are diagnosed based on timing of occurrence in pregnancy (ie, which trimester of pregnancy), symptoms associated with

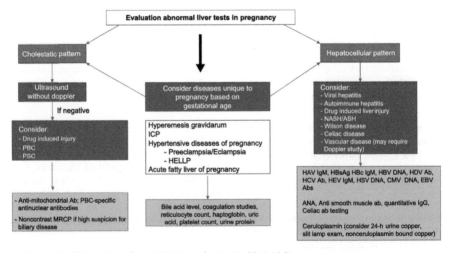

Reprinted with Permission from AASLD Reproductive Health Guidelines

Fig. 1. Diagnostic approach to liver disease in pregnancy.

presentations, as well as pattern of liver test abnormalities. Clinical presentation and management are summarized below. Although they are considered "unique to pregnancy," emerging data suggest that some of these conditions may be associated with chronic liver disease (**Table 1**).

Hyperemesis Gravidarum

Nausea and vomiting in pregnancy (NVP) are common health problems of early pregnancy with a reported prevalence of 75%.[6] Hyperemesis gravidarum (HG) is a severe form of NVP that is characterized by intractable nausea and vomiting, affecting 0.3% to 2% of pregnancies.[6] **Box 1** describes the diagnostic criteria for HG.

It is most common in the first trimester, usually starting at 4 or 5 weeks, and rarely persisting beyond 20 weeks.[7] Risk factors include young age, personal or family history of HG, history of psychiatric illness, nulliparity, and multiple gestations. Proposed hypotheses on the pathophysiology include metabolic and hormonal factors, GI dysmotility, *Helicobacter pylori* infection, and GDF15-GFRAL axis activation.[8–11]

Common laboratory abnormalities include electrolytes derangements, ketosis, metabolic alkalosis, polycythemia, and abnormal liver enzymes. Liver test elevation occurs in almost 50% of patients with HG.[12] Current evidence points toward a possible multifactorial interplay between starvation injury, placental release of inflammatory cytokines, and impairment of fatty acid oxidation in the pathogenesis of liver injury seen in HG.[13] Aminotransferase elevation of up to 200 U/L is the most common biochemical abnormality.[12] There is a propensity for alanine aminotransferase (ALT) to increase more than aspartate aminotransferase (AST) for unclear reasons and mild hyperbilirubinemia can be seen in some cases. The liver synthetic functions remain. Liver imaging is unremarkable but usually done to rule out other causes. Biopsy is rarely indicated except when the diagnosis is uncertain or in cases with atypical increase of liver enzymes. If performed, it is mostly normal, shows steatosis or bland cholestasis.[14]

Treatment of HG is usually supportive regardless of the presence of liver dysfunction. Patients with HG almost always require admission for the administration of intravenous fluids, thiamine, folic acid, and antiemetics. Although maternal–fetal outcomes for mild NVP are generally favorable, HG is associated with a higher incidence of preterm labor, low birth weight, and small gestational age if left untreated.[6] There are no long-term sequelae of liver dysfunction, and the biochemical abnormalities usually correct after cessation of vomiting.[12]

Intrahepatic Cholestasis of Pregnancy

Intrahepatic cholestasis of pregnancy (ICP) is the most common liver disease unique to pregnancy. Occurring in the second and third trimesters, the prevalence in the United States is estimated to be ranging from 0.3% to 5.6%.[15] It is characterized by intense pruritis and elevated serum bile acids with resolution of symptoms after delivery. Risk factors include advanced maternal age, previous history of ICP, multiparity, metabolic syndrome, hepatitis C virus (HCV), and family history of ICP.[16]

The cause of ICP is multifactorial and involves an interplay between genetic, hormonal, and environmental factors. Genetic predisposition likely explains the familial clustering of ICP and recurrence of ICP in future pregnancies. The presence of mutations in biliary transport proteins such as the bile salt export protein pump (BSEP/ABCB11), multidug resistance protein 3 (MDR3/ABCB4), *FIC1* gene (*ATP8B1*), and the *FXR* gene (*NR1H4*) are most cited but still uncommon.[17] ICP onset is most common in the third trimester when estrogen and progesterone serum concentrations are

Table 1
Summary of liver disease unique to pregnancy and their association with other medical conditions

Trimester	Clinical Features	Likely Diagnosis	Association with Other Chronic Disease	
			Preexisting	Postpartum
First	Vomiting, Weight loss, dehydration Laboratories: Aminotransferase—1–5×, Bilirubin <4 mg/dL, Bile acids: Normal Imaging: Mostly normal Biopsy: Mostly normal Treatment: Supportive	HG	NA	NA
Second/Third	Pruritis, Fatigue Laboratories: Aminotransferase—1–5×, Bilirubin <4 mg/dL, Bile acids: 30–100× Imaging: Mostly normal Biopsy: Hepatocellular bile and Canalicular bile plugs Treatment: Urso deoxycholic Acid. Delivery at 37 wk	ICP	Cholecystitis Choledocholithiasis	NAFLD PBC Gallstone Cholecystitis Biliary tree Cancer Liver Cancer
Second/Third/Postpartum	Hypertension, Proteinuria, headache Laboratories: Aminotransferase—1–100×, Bilirubin↑, LDH↑, Platelets↓ Imaging: hepatic infarcts, hematoma, rupture Biopsy: periportal hemorrhage and fibrin deposition Treatment: Supportive, early delivery. Hepatic artery embolization or surgery for expanding hematoma	Preeclampsia/HELLP	Hepatitis C	Heart and cerebral vascular disease
Third/Postpartum	Abdominal pain, hypertension, polydipsia, encephalopathy Laboratories: Aminotransferases—5–10×, Bilirubin↑, Uric acid↑, Platelets↓ Imaging: Steatosis, bright liver Biopsy: Microvesicular steatosis Treatment: Supportive, early delivery. Plasmapheresis	AFLP	NA	NA

Box 1
Diagnostic criteria for Hyperemesis Gravidarum

- Persistent nausea and vomiting
- Laboratory markers of starvation, such as ketonuria
- Weight loss[a]

[a]At least 5% of the prepregnancy weight.[1]

---

high. Some women with a history of ICP may also develop symptoms with the use of oral contraceptive pills.[18]

The classic symptom is itching, most severe in the palms and soles *without* an accompanying rash; however, some also experience epigastric pain, fatigue, and anorexia. Jaundice is very rare although reported late in the disease. Biochemical abnormalities include elevation in bile acid levels, typically greater than 10 μmol/L, with 2-fold to 10-fold increase in aminotransferases. Bilirubin is normal in most cases and alkaline phosphates level may increase but is of limited diagnostic value.[15] Cholelithiasis, cholecystitis, and choledocholithiasis are reported to occur more frequently in patients with ICP and abdominal ultrasound is usually performed to rule out these disorders. Liver biopsy is rarely required and if done shows bile plugs in hepatocytes and canaliculi, predominantly zone 3.[14]

As a rule, pruritis resolves within days after delivery and biochemical abnormalities normalize within weeks. The maternal prognosis is usually favorable. Given association with chronic liver disease[19] (see **Table 1**), genetic testing should be considered in women with severe ICP (total bile acids >100 μmol), recurrent ICP, or early-onset ICP.

Associated fetal risks include preterm births, meconium-stained amniotic fluids, neonatal respiratory depression and asphyxia, and fetal death. These risks increase with increasing bile acid levels and most commonly occur when serum bile acid level is greater than 40 μmol/L.[15] Proposed mechanisms include cardiotoxic effects of bile acids and vasoconstrictive effects of bile acids on placental veins.[18] Therefore, the American College of Obstetricians and Gynecologists recommends delivery at 36 to 37 weeks or at diagnosis if diagnosed after 37 weeks.[20]

Ursodeoxycholic acid (UDCA) is the preferred treatment and earlier studies supported its efficacy in reducing both maternal symptoms and decreasing perinatal morbidity and mortality. However, in the last 3 years, 2 studies have questioned its role. A randomized controlled trial(RCT)by Chappell and colleagues, comparing UDCA 500 mg twice a day with placebo for treatment of ICP, did not reduce any perinatal outcomes.[21] There was a small, statistically significant improvement in itch score but it is unlikely to be clinically relevant. In addition, a meta-analysis did not support the efficacy of UDCA in reducing adverse fetal outcomes.[22] Given the safety profile of UDCA and lack of other therapy, UDCA remains first-line therapy. Other treatments such as rifampicin, cholestyramine, and S-adenosyl-L-methionine (SAMe) have been suggested but lack evidence.[22] Currently, an RTC is being conducted, comparing the effectiveness of UDCA to rifampin in pruritis in early-onset ICP.[23] New mechanisms of action are also being investigated for the treatment of ICP.[24]

Preeclampsia, Eclampsia and Hemolysis, Elevated Liver Enzymes, and Low Platelets Syndrome

The preeclampsia spectrum of disease reflects an overlap among preeclampsia, hemolysis, elevated liver enzymes, and low platelets (HELLP), and even acute fatty liver of pregnancy (AFLP), and therefore may pose a diagnostic challenge in its presentation. Preeclampsia is a multisystem disorder characterized by new-onset hypertension, with additional maternal organ dysfunction after 20 weeks of gestation. Signs and symptoms seen are summarized in **Box 2**. Proteinuria is often present but is not required for diagnosis in presence of other end-organ damage (renal, hepatic, neurologic, or hematologic).[25] Eclampsia is diagnosed when preeclampsia is complicated by seizures. HELLP syndrome, an acronym coined in 1982, is characterized by hemolysis, elevated liver enzymes, and low platelets. It is considered a severe manifestation of the preeclampsia/eclampsia spectrum but can occur in the absence of preexisting preeclampsia. It is estimated that preeclampsia complicates 3% to 5% of pregnancies globally.[26] HELLP syndrome can complicate up to 2% of preeclampsia cases.[12] Risk factors include personal or family history of preeclampsia/HELLP, chronic hypertension, preexisting diabetes, autoimmune disease, and multifetal gestation among others.[25]

Although preeclampsia typically occurs in the second trimester ($\geq$20 weeks of gestation), it is recognized in about 5% of patients postpartum, usually within 48 hours of birth. HELLP, however, typically presents between 28 and 36 weeks of gestation, and almost 30% manifest symptoms in the first week postpartum.[25] The pathophysiology of preeclampsia/eclampsia/HELLP is thought to start early in pregnancy with abnormal placental implantation and decreased perfusion of the placenta as pregnancy progresses. This leads to the release of antiangiogenic factors into the maternal circulation, which interacts with endothelial grown factors and placental growth factors resulting in maternal vascular inflammation, platelet aggregation, and endothelial dysfunction. Liver involvement in hypertensive diseases of the pregnancy is hypothesized to occur secondary to fibrin deposition within the hepatic sinusoids resulting in sinusoidal obstruction and subsequent hepatic ischemia.[12] In preeclampsia, aminotransferases elevation to more than twice the upper limit of normal signifies severe features and parallels the risk of adverse maternal outcomes.[21]

In severe cases, patients can develop hematoma beneath the Glisson Capsule, which has an increased risk for rupture. In HELLP, serum aminotransferases may be elevated more than 10 times the upper limit of normal, and jaundice, if present, is due to hemolysis. Apart from elevated liver function tests (LFTs), other severe hepatic manifestations in HELLP syndrome include hepatic infarction, hemorrhage, and hematoma rupture, which can occur in up to 45% of patients.[12]

Cross-sectional imaging (computerized tomography/MRI) is recommended in preeclampsia/HELLP syndrome, especially in those with abdominal pain, shoulder pain, and hypotension to exclude hemorrhage, rupture, or infarction.[12] A liver biopsy is not required for the diagnosis but if done shows periportal hemorrhage and fibrin

---

Box 2
Signs and symptom of preeclampsia/HELLP syndrome

Clinical Symptoms	Biochemical Abnormalities
• Headache	• Thrombocytopenia
• Vomiting	• Renal insufficiency
• Peripheral edema	• Elevated liver enzymes[a]
• Right upper quadrant pain	
• Vision abnormalities	

[a] Liver enzyme elevation occurs in about 30% of cases in preeclampsia[8]

deposition.[14] Diagnostic criteria have been developed to distinguish HELLP syndrome from preeclampsia/eclampsia spectrum (**Box 3**).

Maternal–fetal complications include preterm labor, postpartum hemorrhage, intrauterine growth retardation, intrauterine death, and prematurity.[25] Studies have also shown that women with preeclampsia and eclampsia have increased risk of heart and cerebral vascular disease later in life.[27]

Management of preeclampsia/eclampsia is supportive and includes administration of antihypertensives, and steroids to improve platelet counts. The only definitive cure is delivery, which is recommended at 37 weeks for preeclampsia, 34 weeks for preeclampsia with severe features, and as soon as possible for eclampsia regardless of gestational age.[25] Studies have demonstrated prophylactic role of aspirin in reducing fetal adverse outcomes in patients with high-risk factors for preeclampsia.[28] Mississippi protocol, which involves administration of magnesium sulfate, corticosteroids, and systolic blood pressure control, has shown to inhibit HELLP syndrome progression.[29] Surgical intervention or hepatic artery embolization is warranted for increasing subcapsular hematoma or hepatic rupture.[12]

Acute Fatty Liver Disease of Pregnancy

AFLP is a rare obstetric emergency characterized by maternal hepatic dysfunction/failure, which can be fatal for both mother and the baby.[30] It usually occurs in the third trimester although 20% present postpartum.[12] It is characterized by maternal microvascular fat deposition in the hepatocytes leading to multiorgan failure. Risk factors include nulliparity, male infants, and twin pregnancies.[30]

Our current understanding of the pathophysiology for AFLP involves a defect in the mitochondrial fatty acid oxidation in the mother and the fetus. The most linked enzyme is long-chain 3-hydroxy acyl-coenzyme A dehydrogenase (LCHAD) deficiency, although other fetal fatty acid oxidation disorders are described.[31,32] A heterozygous mother for a hydroxyacyl-CoA dehydrogenase mutation carrying a fetus with homozygous or compound heterozygous mutation results in the accumulation of hepatotoxic long-chain 3-hydro-fatty acyl metabolites in the maternal circulation and liver.

Initial clinical features are nonspecific with nausea, vomiting, jaundice, and abdominal pain. It can rapidly progress to liver and multiorgan failure including encephalopathy, coagulopathy, pancreatitis, and acute kidney injury (AKI).[12] Biochemical abnormalities include elevation in serum transaminases, hyperbilirubinemia, renal dysfunction, thrombocytopenia, hyperammonemia, and lactic acidosis. The synthetic

---

Box 3
Mississippi classification and Tennessee classification

Mississippi Classification	Tennessee Classification
Class 1:	Complete syndrome:
Platelets <50,000/mm³	Platelets <100,000/mm³
AST or ALT >70 units/L	AST >70 units/L
Lactate dehydrogenase (LDH) >600 units	LDH >600 units/L
Class 2:	
Platelets 50,000–100,000/mm³	Incomplete syndrome:
AST or ALT >70 units/L	Any one or two of the above
LDH >600 units	
Class 3:	
Platelets >100,000/mm³	
AST or ALT >40 units/L	
LDH >600 units	

function of the liver is affected leading to coagulation disorders. Disseminated intra-vascular coagulation complicates 10% of cases.[12] The "Swansea Criteria" has been demonstrated to have 100% sensitivity and 85% positive predictive value in the diag-nosis of AFLP (**Box 4**).[3] Liver imaging shows fatty infiltration and biopsy, if done, shows microvascular fat deposition in the pericentral zone with periportal sparing.[14]

The maternal mortality rate of AFLP in the past was reported to be as high as 90%; however, given our better understanding of the disease and advances in intensive care, maternal mortality now is reported to be around 7% to 18%. Early delivery has improved fetal prognosis but mortality remains substantial at 9% to 23%.[33] Most Patients recover completely; however, severe refractory cases will require liver transplantation.[34] Approximately 20% of women who develop AFLP carry LCHAD-deficient fetuses. Thus, monitoring the offspring of women who develop AFLP at birth for symptoms is recommended. Testing for the mutation can be done in symptomatic infants. Early recognition with rapid delivery is the cornerstone of management, fol-lowed by supportive therapy to the mother and fetus.[33] Therapeutic plasma exchange has also been reported to be beneficial.[35]

CHRONIC LIVER DISEASE IN PREGNANCY

Pregnancy represents a unique opportunity to identify chronic conditions and connect individuals to multidisciplinary management or outpatient follow-up. Screening for hepatitis B virus (HBV) and HCV is now recommended in every pregnancy; however, given the increasing prevalence of NAFLD and alcohol-associated liver disease, these injuries are also common in women of childbearing age. It is imperative to screen women with chronic liver disease (CLD) for fibrosis as portal hypertension (PHT) will worsen during pregnancy and significant increases maternal/fetal risk.

Hepatitis B

HBV infection acquired in adulthood is spontaneously cleared in more than 90% of healthy immunocompetent adults. However, infants who are infected via mother-to-child transmission (MTCT) have a 90% risk of developing chronic hepatitis B (CHB) infection without active/passive immunization. MTCT is responsible for about 50% of the global disease burden of CHB.[36] The peripartum period is the primary risk period for MTCT.[37]

Box 4
Swansea criteria for acute fatty liver of pregnancy

Clinical Features	Laboratory Features
• Nausea and vomiting	• Bilirubin >0.8 mg/dL
• Abdominal pain	• Hypoglycemic <72 mg/dL
• Polydipsia/polyuria	• Leukocytosis >11
• Encephalopathy	• AST or ALT >42 units/L
Radiography Features	• AKI or Creatinine >1.7 mg/dL
• Ascites or echogenic liver	• Coagulopathy or PT > 14 s
Histologic Features	• Ammonia >74 μmol/L
• Microvascular steatosis on liver biopsy	• Uric acid >340 μmol/L

Six or more of the above features are required for diagnosis in absence of another cause.*Ab-breviations:* ALT, alanine aminotransferase; AST, aspartate aminotransferase; PT, prothrombin time.

Fig. 2 describes the approach to antiviral therapy during pregnancy. For women who meet guidelines for HBV treatment (increased ALT and high viral load or concerns for fibrosis), HBV treatment should be initiated during pregnancy.[2] For mothers who do not otherwise meet criteria for antiviral therapy who have HBV DNA is greater than 200,000 IU/mL, antiviral prophylaxis should be initiated at 28 to 32 weeks of gestation for adequate suppression of viral load and prevention of MTCT.[37] For HBV DNA levels of 7-log IU/mL or greater, there should be consideration of earlier treatment to ensure adequate time to reach HBV-DNA levels less than 200,000 IU/mL at delivery.[38]

Given low resistance, high efficacy, and safety in pregnancy, tenofovir disoproxil fumarate is preferred,[2] although there is increasing data for the use of tenofovir alafenamide for HBV in pregnancy.[39] HBV flares have been reported during pregnancy and postpartum following discontinuation of antivirals. Although most are asymptomatic, jaundice, hepatic decompensation, and pregnancy complications have been reported.[40] If antiviral therapy was used solely to prevent MTCT, treatment can be discontinued at delivery or during the first 3 months postpartum. There is a risk for postpartum flare irrespective of if treatment was given or when treatment is stopped. Monitoring is imperative during the first 6 months after birth and treatment discontinuation.[41] Cesarean delivery has not been shown to reduce the risk of MTCT and is not indicated unless required for obstetric indications. Amniocentesis may increase MTCT risk, especially in women with viral load 7-log IU/mL or greater.[2]

After delivery, infants born to hepatitis B surface antigen (HBsAg)-positive mothers should receive the hepatitis B vaccine and hepatitis B immunoglobulin (HBIG) within 12 hours of birth (**Fig. 3**). Breastfeeding is encouraged. At age 9 to 12 months, infants should receive after vaccination serologic testing for HBsAg and anti-HBs. If HBsAg-positive, infants should be referred for appropriate follow-up.[42]

There is conflicting data regarding the influence of HBV infection on pregnancy outcomes (**Table 2** for summary of association of chronic liver diseases with pregnancy outcomes and **Table 3** for summary of association with fetal outcomes). Maternal outcomes including an increased risk of gestational diabetes mellitus (GDM) and antepartum hemorrhage have been reported.[43] HBV infection has been associated with a decreased risk of preeclampsia, particularly in the Asian population.[44] Preterm births, stillbirths, and spontaneous abortions have also been reported in pregnant women with HBV infection.[43] A recent systematic review and meta-analysis by Jiang and colleagues demonstrated a higher risk of ICP among HBV-positive mothers and an increased risk of HBV infection among patients with ICP. Given these findings, they suggest screening for HBV infection among pregnant women with ICP.[45]

Hepatitis C

HCV infection diagnosed during pregnancy has increased, particularly due to intravenous drug use and the opioid epidemic.[46] The rate of maternal HCV infection increased from 1.8 cases per 1000 live births to 4.7 cases per 1000 live births in the United States.[47] The AASLD recommends universal screening for HCV infection during each pregnancy with an anti-HCV antibody test, and those with positive results should be referred to a specialist for the evaluation of antiviral therapy after completion of pregnancy and breastfeeding.[2] More recently, the center for disease control and prevention (CDC), the United States preventive services task force (USPSTF), and American College of obstetricians and gynecologists (ACOG) have all also endorsed universal screening for HCV during pregnancy.

Understanding the risk of MTCT of HCV and association of HCV with pregnancy outcomes is important in counseling women. The rate of MTCT, which can occur

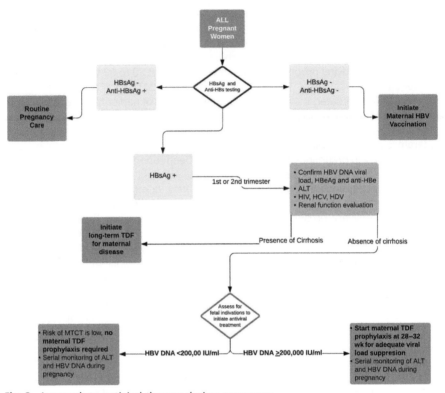

Fig. 2. Approach to antiviral therapy during pregnancy.

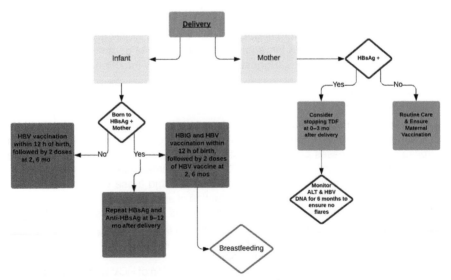

Fig. 3. Approach to infants born to HBsAg-positive mothers.

Table 2
Summary of effect of chronic liver diseases in pregnancy on the risk of maternal outcomes

Disease	Infertility	GDM	IPC	Hypertensive Disorders of Pregnancy
HBV	No change in risk	Increased	Increased	Decreased
HCV	No change in risk	Increased	Increased	No known change in risk
Cirrhosis	Increased	No change in risk	Increased	Increased
NAFLD	No change in risk[a]	Increased	No known change in risk	Increased
AIH	No known change in risk	Increased	No known change in risk	Increased
WD	Increased	No change in risk	No known change in risk	No known change in risk
PBC	No known change in risk	No known change in risk	No known change in risk	No known change in risk
PSC	No known change in risk	No known change in risk	No known change in risk	No known change in risk

[a] In the absence of concomitant PCOS.

intrapartum, peripartum, or postpartum (most common), has been estimated to be 5.8% in mothers with HCV viremia and 10.8% in mothers with HCV–human immunodeficiency virus (HIV) coinfection.[48] Other than HIV suppression in HIV/HCV-coinfected women, there are no known interventions to decrease the risk of MTCT of HCV.[46] There may be passive transfer of HCV antibody from MTCT, which can

Table 3
Summary of effect of chronic liver diseases in pregnancy on the risk of fetal outcomes

Disease	Spontaneous Abortion	Preterm Birth	Stillbirth	Risk of MTCT
HBV	Increased	Increased	Increased	HBeAg (−): 10%–40% HBeAg (+): 70%–90%
HCV	No known change in risk	Increased	No known change in risk	5.8%
Cirrhosis	Increased	Increased	Increased	N/A
NAFLD	Increased	Increased	No known change in risk	N/A
AIH	Increased	Increased	No known change in risk	N/A
WD	Increased	No known change in risk	Increased	N/A
PBC	No known change in risk	Increased	No change in risk	N/A
PSC	No known change in risk	Increased	No change in risk	N/A

Table 4
Breastfeeding recommendations in chronic liver diseases

Disease	Recommendation
HCV	Safe *unless* skin breakdown with bleeding is present or treatment with antiviral therapy is ongoing
HBV	Safe even if cracked or bleeding nipples because infants are protected by vaccination and HBIG
Cirrhosis	Safe[a]
NAFLD	Safe
AIH	Safe
WD	Not recommended
PBC	Safe only if UDCA used as treatment option
PSC	Safe only if UDCA used as treatment option

[a] Adequate protein intake is encouraged.

remain for up to 18 months, thus recommendations suggest that these children should be tested for anti-HCV after 18 months of age and subsequently with HCV-RNA to confirm viremia.[49] In order to decrease the risk of MTCT, avoiding invasive fetal monitoring, episiotomy, and prolonged rupture of the membranes is recommended. If invasive prenatal testing is required, amniocentesis is favored over chorionic villus sampling and fetal blood sampling. Neither the mode of delivery nor breastfeeding influence the risk of MTCT.[50,51] Breastfeeding is recommended, unless skin breakdown with bleeding is present or treatment with antiviral therapy is ongoing[2] (**Table 4**). **Box 5** summarizes current data on association of HCV with adverse pregnancy outcomes.

Treatment of hepatitis is generally encouraged prepregnancy or postpartum. If treatment is delayed, HCV polymerase chain reaction (PCR) testing should be performed before therapy because there are reports of spontaneous clearance after pregnancy. If treatment postpartum is desired, confirmation HCV-RNA before postpartum treatment is recommended.[2,55] The safety and efficacy of direct-acting antivirals during pregnancy is currently being evaluated.[56] Although previously recommended to avoid any treatment during pregnancy, current recommendations suggest treatment considerations on an individual basis after a risk and benefit discussion between provider and patient. Discussions should include the risk of MTCT, risk for virologic relapse, finances, patient preferences, and limited safety data.

Box 5
HCV impact on maternal and fetal outcomes

- Higher rates of preterm birth, small for gestational age, low birth weight, and intrauterine fetal death.[52]

- A 20-fold increased risk of ICP compared with non-HCV pregnant women.[53] Bile acids should be checked in HCV-positive mothers with pruritus and HCV-antibody should be checked in women with ICP.

- Reports of increased rates of antepartum hemorrhage, GDM, postpartum hemorrhage and premature rupture of membranes.[54]

- Course of HCV infection is not affected by pregnancy; no specific monitoring is required.[2]

Nonalcoholic Fatty Liver Disease

NAFLD is the most common chronic liver disease found in women of childbearing age.[57] Physiologic changes of pregnancy including increased adipose tissue, decreased insulin sensitivity, and increased lipolysis may increase the metabolic risks of women with NAFLD.[2] NAFLD has been associated with maternal complications including GDM, postpartum hemorrhage,[2,58,59] and gestational hypertension[59] (see **Table 2**). An increased risk of fetal outcomes such as preterm births and large for gestational birth has also been found in pregnant patients with NAFLD.[59] A recent systematic review found a novel association between pregnant NAFLD patients and a history of prior miscarriage or abortion, thought to be related to obesity.[59] Given the high incidence of adverse maternal and fetal outcomes in pregnant patients with NAFLD, preconception counseling should include a review of the potential risks associated with pregnancy in NAFLD in addition to counseling about the benefits of weight optimization and metabolic comorbidities before conception.[2] Breastfeeding is encouraged in NAFLD patients because lactation decreases maternal lipid, glucose, and insulin levels while improving insulin sensitivity. A longer duration of lactation has been associated with a lower rate of future NAFLD among offspring and a lower incidence of maternal metabolic complications including NAFLD, increased postpartum weight loss, and a reduction in heart disease and diabetes.[2,60,61] Although there are no NAFLD-specific medications are approved for use in or after pregnancy, management of NAFLD in pregnancy is focused on preventing excess weight gain, close monitoring of fetal growth, monitoring of liver tests similar to nonpregnant women, treatment of metabolic comorbidities, and lifestyle modifications to achieve an optimal weight.[2] Given the risk of disease progression, follow-up with a provider experienced in NAFLD management should be encouraged postpartum.

Autoimmune Hepatitis

Autoimmune hepatitis (AIH) is a chronic inflammatory liver disease that can progress to cirrhosis if left untreated.[62] Patients with known and undertreated AIH may have an increased risk of pregnancy-related complications. The evaluation and diagnosis in the pregnant patient is similar to that of a nonpregnant patient.[2] Histology may be required in disease staging and help guide clinical management, especially in patients who lack atypical findings, negative autoantibodies, and or immunoglobulin G levels.[63] There may be a moderately increased risk of preterm birth and small for gestational age with liver biopsy, thus a discussion with the mother regarding risks weighed against the advantages of obtaining a liver biopsy is important.[64] About 20% of patients with AIH will flare during pregnancy,[65] thus AASLD recommends that conception should be delayed for at least 1 year after a stable dose of immunosuppression is maintained. Liver enzymes should be monitored during each trimester and every 2 to 4 weeks for at least 6 months postpartum due to the high rates of flares and relapse, respectively.[2,66] AIH has been associated with an increased risk of preterm birth, small for gestational age children,[67,68] spontaneous abortions,[1,66] GDM,[69] and hypertensive complications including preeclampsia, eclampsia, and/or hemolysis, elevated liver enzymes, low platelets (HELLP)[62] (see **Tables 2** and **3**). According to AASLD, patients with AIH should be counseled regarding the potential risks of treatments including azathioprine and 6-mercaptopurine (6-MP) but these drugs are safe in pregnancy and lactation.[2,62] Steroids indicated for treatment of AIH, prednisone and budesonide, are considered low risk in pregnancy and lactation. Mycophenolic acid (MPA) is contraindicated in pregnancy and lactation due to high risk of congenital malformations and spontaneous abortions. MPA should be discontinued 6 weeks before conception attempts, and a negative pregnancy test is required within 1 week of starting treatment with MPA.[2,70] Breastfeeding is safe.[2]

Wilson Disease

Wilson disease (WD) is an autosomal recessive disorder associated with a mutation on the P-type aminophospholipid transporter synthase ATP7B transmembrane copper carrier, resulting in excess copper deposition, especially in the liver and brain.[71] Due to expression of ATP7B in the placenta, uterus and ovaries, there are effects of excess copper on pregnancy outcomes such as higher rates of infertility, stillbirth, and spontaneous abortions[2,71] (see **Tables 2** and **3**). Thus, women with WD should be enrolled in genetic counseling and medication safety regarding various treatment options needs to be discussed. AASLD recommends dose reduction of chelating agents including ᴅ-penicillamine and trientine by 25% to 50% of the prepregnancy dose due to the risk of fetal teratogenicity.[2,72] Zinc dosage can be safely maintained throughout pregnancy,[73] although a recent case series demonstrated birth defects with zinc usage in pregnancy raising the possibility that this treatment's safety profile needs to be further evaluated.[71] During pregnancy, close monitoring of copper levels is necessary to avoid over chelation during pregnancy because this may adversely affect the fetus.[2] If treatment is discontinued during pregnancy, there is a high risk of maternal liver failure, WD flares, and copper deposition in placenta with subsequent fetal damage.[1] After delivery, chelating agents require uptitration to prepregnancy doses and breastfeeding is associated with infant risks as all WD drugs are excreted in breast milk, raising potential of copper deficiency in the infant. For these reasons, breastfeeding is not recommended for mothers with WD.[2,74]

Primary Biliary Cholangitis

Primary biliary cholangitis (PBC) is a chronic, autoimmune cholestatic liver disease of the intrahepatic bile ducts, predominantly affecting women. Most patients are diagnosed in the sixth decade of life but 25% of patients are of childbearing age at diagnosis,[75] and 33% of new diagnoses are made during pregnancy.[2] Pregnancy in PBC was thought to have poor outcomes[76] but recent literature reports good maternal and fetal outcomes.[75,77] Aminotransferases and total bile acid concentrations are expected to remain normal during pregnancy and an increase in these values may suggest cholestasis.[78] Thus, it is recommended to measure bile acids during pregnancy in those with known PBC, and treat if elevated, particularly in the 40 to 100 range.[2] A recent study suggested that pregnancy in women with PBC and PSC is well tolerated but linked to higher rates of preterm birth, possibly due to high levels of maternal bile acids.[77] Postpartum, 60% to 70% of patients with PBC may have an increase in disease activity,[79] thus close monitoring postpartum is recommended. Immunoglobulin M levels and M2 antibody titers may decline in pregnancy but return to baseline levels postpartum.[2,80] Pruritis is a common symptom of PBC, which may worsen in about 50% of patients with PBC during pregnancy.[79] UDCA is not associated with adverse effects and is recommended for PBC in pregnancy and during breastfeeding.[2,80] Obeticholic acid and fibrates are not recommended during pregnancy and lactation due to insufficient safety data. For the management of pruritis in pregnancy, addition of cholestyramine, rifampin, antihistamines, or SAMe to UDCA may be considered. Vitamin K deficiency may be exacerbated by cholestyramine, thus regular monitoring of prothrombin time (PT) is recommended.[2]

Primary Sclerosing Cholangitis

Primary sclerosing cholangitis (PSC) is a progressive autoimmune, cholestatic liver disease that affects the intrahepatic and extrahepatic bile ducts, leading to fibrosis and cirrhosis.[81] Seventy percent of patients with PSC have concurrent inflammatory bowel disease (IBD),[82] limiting data available on outcomes of pregnant patients without IBD. Although a decrease in fertility has not been linked to PSC,[83] there have been reports of increased rates of preterm births[77,84] and cesarean delivery in these patients.[84] Nonetheless, no differences were seen in small for gestational age, stillbirths, or neonatal deaths.[2,84] Although liver tests remain normal in most patients, up to one-third develop nonclinically significant increased liver tests postpartum.[84] Guidelines suggest consideration of measurement of total serum bile acids in the first trimester. In the event of new-onset or worsening pruritis in pregnancy, comparison of bile acid levels to the first trimester will aid in excluding ICP.[2] No data currently supports a therapeutic benefit of UDCA in PSC[2,85] but pregnant patients on UDCA are more likely to have stable liver enzymes than those who are not.[83] Patients who are taking UDCA before pregnancy can continue throughout their pregnancy because UDCA is considered safe in pregnancy.[77] Patients with PSC who develop new pruritus or worsening liver enzymes during pregnancy should be initially evaluated with ultrasound due to possibility of new stricture formation. Magnetic retrograde cholangiopancreatography can safely be performed in the second and third trimesters but should be avoided in the first trimester. Endoscopic retrograde cholangiopancreatography should be reserved for cases requiring endoscopic therapy.[85] Treatment of pruritus in pregnancy is similar to that of PBC.

Cirrhosis and Portal Hypertension

Fertility is not affected by compensated cirrhosis but will be reduced in those with clinically significant PHT and decompensated cirrhosis, due to hepatocyte injury leading to chronic elevation in estrogen levels and subsequent anovulation.[86] Complications of cirrhosis during pregnancy include worsening PHT and esophageal variceal bleeding.[87] Variceal bleeding is more common in the second trimester of pregnancy and during labor due to increased circulating blood volume and decreased venous return due to gravid uterus pressure on the inferior vena cava.[88] Due to improved care of pregnant women with cirrhosis, PHT and cirrhosis are no longer considered absolute contraindications to pregnancy.[2] The Model for End-Stage Liver Disease (MELD) score has been used to predict risk of significant liver-related complications during pregnancy. A MELD score of 10 or greater predicted liver-related complications with 83% sensitivity and specificity, whereas MELD scores less than 6 predicted positive outcomes with least complications.[89] Still all women with cirrhosis, especially those with MELD 10 or greater or history of prior hepatic decompensation, should be counseled on the potential risk of worsening liver disease during pregnancy.[2]

Portal Hypertension in Pregnancy

One of the most dreaded complications of PHT in pregnant women with cirrhosis is variceal bleeding. Maternal and fetal mortality is high, with a rate of 18% and 11%, respectively.[90] Current guidelines recommend preconception esophagogastroduodenoscopy (EGD) screening for varices within 12 months of conception, even in patients with noncirrhotic PHT (**Fig. 4** for approach to management). A second trimester EGD is recommended in women who do not receive a preconception EGD, have new symptoms of hepatic decompensation, or have an ongoing liver injury (active alcohol use, untreated HCV infection). Nonselective beta blockers (NSBB) are recommended for primary and

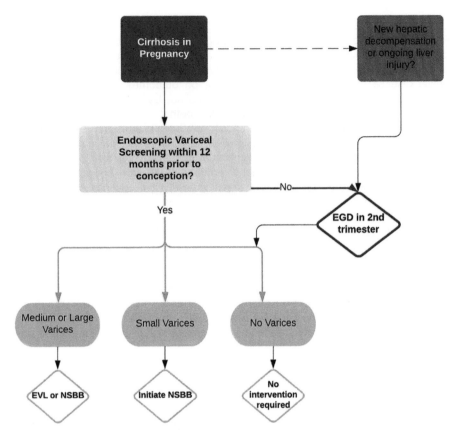

Fig. 4. Approach to PHT in pregnancy.

secondary prophylaxis of bleeding. Propanolol is the favored NSBB in pregnancy. Esophageal variceal ligation (EVL) can be performed on medium or large varices (>5 mm) or if there is evidence of high-risk bleeding stigmata such as a red whale sign or cherry red spots. During EGD in pregnancy, safe anesthetics include propofol, fentanyl, midazolam, and meperidine.[2] Endoscopy is generally safe in pregnancy but the risks and benefits must be reviewed to assess patient readiness for procedure.[1]

Complications of PHT in pregnancy include acute variceal hemorrhage and splenic artery aneurysm (**Fig. 5**). Management of acute variceal hemorrhage in pregnancy is similar to that of nonpregnant individuals.[2] In patients with refractory bleeding despite medical and endoscopic measures, rescue transjugular intrahepatic portosystemic shunt (TIPS) is not contraindicated if refractory bleeding risk is high.[91] Secondary prophylaxis for variceal bleeds include NSBB and EVL, with preference of a combination of therapy.[92] Splenic artery aneurysm rupture is a rare complication that may present as abdominal pain and syncope in the third trimester, with high mortality rates (70%–95%) in both fetus and mother. Management typically includes transcatheter embolization with ligation splenectomy for cases in which embolization fails or is unavailable.[93]

The mode of fetal delivery should only be guided by obstetric indications because there is no benefit to vaginal versus cesarean section.[1,2] Vaginal deliveries carry an increased risk of variceal bleeding because of increased intra-abdominal pressures from stress maneuvers during labor.[94] Cesarean sections are associated with

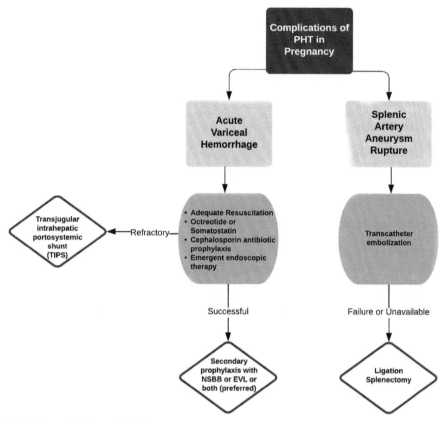

Fig. 5. Complications of PHT in pregnancy.

increased risks of postpartum ascites and bleeding from vessel injury but may be required during fetal distress.[95]

Fetal and Maternal Outcomes of Cirrhosis in Pregnancy

Close monitoring of cirrhotic patients during pregnancy is important as complications may result in high morbidity and mortality. Management in a multidisciplinary center with maternal fetal medicine and gastroenterology/hepatology is recommended.[1] Although mortality was previously thought to be high in these patients, newer studies report rates less than 2%.[96] Data from the United States Nationwide Inpatient Sample revealed hepatic decompensation in 15% of pregnant women with cirrhosis, ascites in 11% and variceal bleed in 5%.[90] A recent population-based study identified increased rates of ICP, puerperal infections, preterm births, large for gestational age infants and neonatal respiratory distress among women with cirrhosis.[96] Pregnancy in cirrhosis has also been associated with higher risks of cesarean delivery, placenta abruptae, and gestational hypertension.[90] Spontaneous abortion and stillbirth has been reported to be more common in women with cirrhosis.[97]

LIVER DISEASE COINCIDENTAL TO PREGNANCY

Evaluation of the patient with liver disease in pregnancy should also address potential liver disease "coincidental to pregnancy." This includes acute viral hepatitis (including hepatitis A virus [HAV], hepatitis E virus [HEV], and herpes simplex virus [HSV]) that may present during pregnancy, biliary disease (ie, gallstones, which have increased incidence of complications in pregnancy), as well as liver lesions. Management of acute viral hepatitis is largely supportive although may be associated with a more severe course in pregnancy particularly with HEV. Ultrasound should be performed in the evaluation of abnormal liver tests, most notably if associated with other symptoms such as abdominal pain, to assess for gallstones, and evidence of cholecystitis should prompt surgical evaluation. Finally, although most liver lesions can be safely monitored in pregnancy, adenomas greater than 5 cm are associated with increases in size in pregnancy and potential rupture.[2] Ideally address before pregnancy with embolization or resection, large lesions require intervention and close follow-up with imaging during each trimester is recommended irrespective of size.

SUMMARY

Liver disease in pregnancy represents a broad spectrum of liver pathologic condition and liver-related conditions that require early recognition in order to guide care. Evaluation requires judicious testing to exclude chronic liver disease, coincidental liver injury, and pregnancy specific liver injury. Early recognition and management of liver disease in pregnancy is crucial in order to optimize maternal and fetal outcomes, as well as to link patients to liver specialists and possible ongoing care after delivery if indicated.

CLINICS CARE POINTS

- Evaluation of liver injury in pregnancy should include a comprehensive evaluation for underlying liver disease as well as consideration for liver disease unique to pregnancy.
- Symptoms of Hyperemesis gravidarum and ICP resolve during pregnancy and at delivery, respectively.
- Treatment of AFLP and HELLP is with urgent delivery.
- Ursodiol is the treatment of choice for ICP.
- All pregnant individuals should be screened for hepatitis B and for hepatitis.
- Treatment of hepatitis B in pregnancy is determined based on the maternal viral load and disease stage.
- Poor disease control of autoimmune hepatitis is associated with adverse pregnancy outcomes.
- Endoscopic evaluation should occur within 12 months prior to conception in patients with cirrhosis.

DISCLOSURE

G. Karim has no disclosures. D. Giri has no disclosures. T. Kushner has served in advisory role for Gilead, Abbvie. N. Reau has served in advisory role for Gilead, Abbvie.

REFERENCES

1. Tran TT, Ahn J, Reau NS. ACG clinical guideline: liver disease and pregnancy. Am J Gastroenterol 2016;111(2):176–94 [quiz: 196].

2. Sarkar M, Brady CW, Fleckenstein J, et al. Reproductive health and liver disease: Practice guidance by the American association for the study of liver diseases. Hepatology 2021;73(1):318–65.

3. Ch'ng CL, Morgan M, Hainsworth I, et al. Prospective study of liver dysfunction in pregnancy in Southwest Wales. Gut 2002;51(6):876–80.

4. García-Romero CS, Guzman C, Cervantes A, et al. Liver disease in pregnancy: medical aspects and their implications for mother and child. Ann Hepatol 2019;18(4):553–62.

5. Ellington SR, Flowers L, Legardy-Williams JK, et al. Recent trends in hepatic diseases during pregnancy in the United States, 2002-2010. Am J Obstet Gynecol 2015;212(4):524 e1–7.

6. Goodwin TM. Hyperemesis gravidarum. Obstet Gynecol Clin North Am 2008; 35(3):401–17, viii.

7. Jarvis S, Nelson-Piercy C. Management of nausea and vomiting in pregnancy. Bmj 2011;342:d3606.

8. Fejzo MS, Arzy D, Tian R, et al. Evidence GDF15 Plays a role in familial and recurrent hyperemesis gravidarum. Geburtshilfe Frauenheilkd 2018;78(9):866–70.

9. Fejzo MS, Ingles SA, Wilson M, et al. High prevalence of severe nausea and vomiting of pregnancy and hyperemesis gravidarum among relatives of affected individuals. Eur J Obstet Gynecol Reprod Biol 2008;141(1):13–7.

10. Golberg D, Szilagyi A, Graves L. Hyperemesis gravidarum and Helicobacter pylori infection: a systematic review. Obstet Gynecol 2007;110(3):695–703.

11. Verberg MFG, Gillott DJ, Al-Fardan N, et al. Hyperemesis gravidarum, a literature review. Hum Reprod Update 2005;11(5):527–39.

12. Westbrook RH, Dusheiko G, Williamson C. Pregnancy and liver disease. J Hepatol 2016;64(4):933–45.

13. Outlaw WM, Ibdah JA, Koch KL. Hyperemesis Gravidarum and Maternal Liver Disease. Madame Curie Bioscience Database [Internet]. Landes Bioscience; 2013.

14. Rolfes DB, Ishak KG. Liver disease in pregnancy. Histopathology 1986;10(6): 555–70.

15. Geenes V, Williamson C. Intrahepatic cholestasis of pregnancy. World J Gastroenterol 2009;15(17):2049–66.

16. Bicocca MJ, Sperling JD, Chauhan SP. Intrahepatic cholestasis of pregnancy: review of six national and regional guidelines. Eur J Obstet Gynecol Reprod Biol 2018;231:180–7.

17. Dixon PH, Sambrotta M, Chambers J, et al. An expanded role for heterozygous mutations of ABCB4, ABCB11, ATP8B1, ABCC2 and TJP2 in intrahepatic cholestasis of pregnancy. Sci Rep 2017;7(1):11823.

18. Ovadia C, Williamson C. Intrahepatic cholestasis of pregnancy: recent advances. Clin Dermatol 2016;34(3):327–34.

19. Monrose E, Bui A, Rosenbluth E, et al. Burden of future liver abnormalities in patients with intrahepatic cholestasis of pregnancy. Am J Gastroenterol 2021; 116(3):568–75.

20. Kaneuchi Y, Sekiguchi M, Kameda T, et al. Temporal and Spatial changes of mu-opioid Receptors in the Brain, Spinal Cord and Dorsal Root Ganglion in a Rat Lumbar Disc Herniation Model. Spine (Phila Pa 1976) 2019;44(2):85–95.

21. Chappell LC, Bell JL, Smith A, et al. Ursodeoxycholic acid versus placebo in women with intrahepatic cholestasis of pregnancy (PITCHES): a randomised controlled trial. Lancet 2019;394(10201):849–60.

22. Walker KF, Chappell LC, Hague WM, et al. Pharmacological interventions for treating intrahepatic cholestasis of pregnancy. Cochrane Database Syst Rev 2020;7. https://doi.org/10.1002/14651858.CD000493.pub3.

23. Available at: https://www.clinicaltrialsregister.eu/ctr-search/trial/2018-004011-44/Fl. Accessed March 13, 2021.

24. Available at: https://clinicaltrials.gov/ct2/show/NCT04718961. Accessed March 13, 2021.

25. Bradley H, Hall EW, Rosenthal EM, et al. Hepatitis C virus prevalence in 50 U.S. States and D.C. By Sex, birth cohort, and Race: 2013-2016. Hepatol Commun 2020;4(3):355–70.

26. Mol BWJ, Roberts CT, Thangaratinam S, et al. Pre-eclampsia. Lancet 2016; 387(10022):999–1011.

27. Seely EW, Tsigas E, Rich-Edwards JW. Preeclampsia and future cardiovascular disease in women: How good are the data and how can we manage our patients? Semin Perinatol 2015;39(4):276–83.

28. Roberge S, Nicolaides K, Demers S, et al. The role of aspirin dose on the prevention of preeclampsia and fetal growth restriction: systematic review and meta-analysis. Am J Obstet Gynecol 2017;216(2):110–20.e6.

29. Martin JN Jr, Owens MY, Keiser SD, et al. Standardized Mississippi Protocol treatment of 190 patients with HELLP syndrome: slowing disease progression and preventing new major maternal morbidity. Hypertens Pregnancy 2012;31(1):79–90.

30. Knight M, Nelson-Piercy C, Kurinczuk JJ, et al. A prospective national study of acute fatty liver of pregnancy in the UK. Gut 2008;57(7):951–6.

31. Browning MF, Levy HL, Wilkins-Haug LE, et al. Fetal fatty acid oxidation defects and maternal liver disease in pregnancy. Obstet Gynecol 2006;107(1):115–20.

32. Ibdah JA, Bennett MJ, Rinaldo P, et al. A fetal fatty-acid oxidation disorder as a cause of liver disease in pregnant women. N Engl J Med 1999;340(22):1723–31.

33. Hay JE. Liver disease in pregnancy. Hepatology 2008;47(3):1067–76.

34. Kushner T, Tholey D, Dodge J, et al. Outcomes of liver transplantation for acute fatty liver disease of pregnancy. Am J Transplant 2019;19(7):2101–7.

35. Rebahi H, Still ME, El Adib AR. A successful use of therapeutic plasma exchange in a fulminant form of acute fatty liver of pregnancy. J Gynecol Obstet Hum Reprod 2019;48(2):133–7. https://doi.org/10.1016/j.jogoh.2018.10.001.

36. Joshi SS, Coffin CS. Hepatitis B and pregnancy: virologic and Immunologic Characteristics. Hepatol Commun 2020;4(2):157–71.

37. Terrault NA, Levy MT, Cheung KW, et al. Viral hepatitis and pregnancy. Nat Rev Gastroenterol Hepatol 2021;18(2):117–30.

38. Chen HL, Lee CN, Chang CH, et al. Efficacy of maternal tenofovir disoproxil fumarate in interrupting mother-to-infant transmission of hepatitis B virus. Hepatology 2015;62(2):375–86.

39. Chen R, Zou J, Long L, et al. Safety and efficacy of tenofovir alafenamide fumarate in early-Middle pregnancy for mothers with chronic hepatitis B. Front Med (Lausanne) 2021;8:796901.

40. Kushner T, Shaw PA, Kalra A, et al. Incidence, determinants and outcomes of pregnancy-associated hepatitis B flares: a regional hospital-based cohort study. Liver Int 2018;38(5):813–20.

41. Bzowej NH, Tran TT, Li R, et al. Total Alanine aminotransferase (ALT) flares in pregnant North American women with chronic hepatitis B infection: results from a prospective Observational study. Am J Gastroenterol 2019;114(8):1283–91.

42. Schillie S, Vellozzi C, Reingold A, et al. Prevention of hepatitis B virus infection in the United States: recommendations of the advisory Committee on immunization Practices. MMWR Recomm Rep 2018;67(1):1–31.
43. Sirilert S, Tongsong T. Hepatitis B virus infection in pregnancy: Immunological Response, Natural course and pregnancy outcomes. J Clin Med 2021;10(13).
44. Huang QT, Chen JH, Zhong M, et al. Chronic hepatitis B infection is associated with decreased risk of preeclampsia: a meta-analysis of Observational studies. Cell Physiol Biochem 2016;38(5):1860–8.
45. Jiang R, Wang T, Yao Y, et al. Hepatitis B infection and intrahepatic cholestasis of pregnancy: a systematic review and meta-analysis. Medicine (Baltimore) 2020; 99(31):e21416.
46. Kushner T, Reau N. Changing epidemiology, implications, and recommendations for hepatitis C in women of childbearing age and during pregnancy. J Hepatol 2021;74(3):734–41.
47. Rossi RM, Wolfe C, Brokamp R, et al. Reported prevalence of maternal hepatitis C virus infection in the United States. Obstet Gynecol 2020;135(2):387–95.
48. Benova L, Mohamoud YA, Calvert C, et al. Vertical transmission of hepatitis C virus: systematic review and meta-analysis. Clin Infect Dis 2014;59(6):765–73.
49. Hillemanns P, Dannecker C, Kimmig R, et al. Obstetric risks and vertical transmission of hepatitis C virus infection in pregnancy. Acta Obstet Gynecol Scand 2000; 79(7):543–7.
50. Hughes BL, Page CM, Kuller JA. Hepatitis C in pregnancy: screening, treatment, and management. Am J Obstet Gynecol 2017;217(5):B2–12.
51. Cottrell EB, Chou R, Wasson N, et al. Reducing risk for mother-to-infant transmission of hepatitis C virus: a systematic review for the U.S. Preventive Services Task Force. Ann Intern Med 2013;158(2):109–13.
52. Money D, Boucoiran I, Wagner E, et al. Obstetrical and neonatal outcomes among women infected with hepatitis C and their infants. J Obstet Gynaecol Can 2014;36(9):785–94.
53. Wijarnpreecha K, Thongprayoon C, Sanguankeo A, et al. Hepatitis C infection and intrahepatic cholestasis of pregnancy: a systematic review and meta-analysis. Clin Res Hepatol Gastroenterol 2017;41(1):39–45.
54. Rezk M, Omar Z. Deleterious impact of maternal hepatitis-C viral infection on maternal and fetal outcome: a 5-year prospective study. Arch Gynecol Obstet 2017;296(6):1097–102.
55. Hashem M, Jhaveri R, Saleh DA, et al. Spontaneous viral load decline and subsequent clearance of chronic hepatitis C virus in postpartum women Correlates with favorable Interleukin-28B gene Allele. Clin Infect Dis 2017;65(6):999–1005.
56. Chappell CA, Scarsi KK, Kirby BJ, et al. Ledipasvir plus sofosbuvir in pregnant women with hepatitis C virus infection: a phase 1 pharmacokinetic study. Lancet Microbe 2020;1(5):e200–8.
57. Doycheva I, Watt KD, Rifai G, et al. Increasing burden of chronic liver disease among Adolescents and young adults in the USA: a Silent epidemic. Dig Dis Sci 2017;62(5):1373–80.
58. Sarkar M, Djerboua M, Flemming JA. NAFLD cirrhosis is rising among childbearing women and is the most common cause of cirrhosis in pregnancy. Clin Gastroenterol Hepatol 2022;20(2):e315–8.
59. El Jamaly H, Eslick GD, Weltman M. Systematic review with meta-analysis: nonalcoholic fatty liver disease and the association with pregnancy outcomes. Clin Mol Hepatol 2022;28(1):52–66.

60. Ajmera VH, Terrault NA, VanWagner LB, et al. Longer lactation duration is associated with decreased prevalence of non-alcoholic fatty liver disease in women. J Hepatol 2019;70(1):126–32.
61. Gunderson EP, Jacobs DR Jr, Chiang V, et al. Duration of lactation and incidence of the metabolic syndrome in women of reproductive age according to gestational diabetes mellitus status: a 20-Year prospective study in CARDIA (Coronary Artery Risk Development in Young Adults). Diabetes 2010;59(2):495–504.
62. Wang CW, Grab J, Tana MM, et al. Outcomes of pregnancy in autoimmune hepatitis: a population-based study. Hepatology 2022;75(1):5–12.
63. Kothadia JP, Shah JM. Autoimmune hepatitis and pregnancy. Treasure Island, FL: StatPearls. StatPearls Publishing. Copyright © 2022, StatPearls Publishing LLC.; 2022.
64. Ludvigsson JF, Marschall HU, Hagström H, et al. Pregnancy outcome in women undergoing liver biopsy during pregnancy: a nationwide population-based cohort study. Hepatology 2018;68(2):625–33.
65. Peters MG. Management of autoimmune hepatitis in pregnant women. Gastroenterol Hepatol (N Y) 2017;13(8):504–6.
66. Terrabuio DR, Abrantes-Lemos CP, Carrilho FJ, et al. Follow-up of pregnant women with autoimmune hepatitis: the disease behavior along with maternal and fetal outcomes. J Clin Gastroenterol 2009;43(4):350–6.
67. Grønbaek L, Vilstrup H, Jepsen P. Pregnancy and birth outcomes in a Danish nationwide cohort of women with autoimmune hepatitis and matched population controls. Aliment Pharmacol Ther 2018;48(6):655–63.
68. Braga A, Vasconcelos C, Braga J. Autoimmune hepatitis and pregnancy. Best Pract Res Clin Obstet Gynaecol 2020;68:23–31.
69. El Jamaly H, Eslick GD, Weltman M. Systematic review with meta-analysis: autoimmune hepatitis in pregnancy. Scand J Gastroenterol 2021;56(10):1194–204.
70. Kim M, Rostas S, Gabardi S. Mycophenolate fetal toxicity and risk evaluation and mitigation strategies. Am J Transplant 2013;13(6):1383–9.
71. Mussi MCL, Nardelli MJ, Santos BC, et al. Pregnancy outcomes in Wilson's disease women: Single-center case series. Fetal Pediatr Pathol 2021;1–8. https://doi.org/10.1080/15513815.2021.1960940.
72. Pinter R, Hogge WA, McPherson E. Infant with severe penicillamine embryopathy born to a woman with Wilson disease. Am J Med Genet A 2004;128a(3):294–8.
73. Brewer GJ, Johnson VD, Dick RD, et al. Treatment of Wilson's disease with zinc. XVII: treatment during pregnancy. Hepatology 2000;31(2):364–70.
74. Michalczyk A, Bastow E, Greenough M, et al. ATP7B expression in human breast epithelial cells is mediated by lactational hormones. J Histochem Cytochem 2008;56(4):389–99.
75. Trivedi PJ, Kumagi T, Al-Harthy N, et al. Good maternal and fetal outcomes for pregnant women with primary biliary cirrhosis. Clin Gastroenterol Hepatol 2014; 12(7):1179–85.e1.
76. Whelton MJ, Sherlock S. Pregnancy in patients with hepatic cirrhosis. Management and outcome. Lancet 1968;2(7576):995–9.
77. Cauldwell M, Mackie FL, Steer PJ, et al. Pregnancy outcomes in women with primary biliary cholangitis and primary sclerosing cholangitis: a retrospective cohort study. Bjog 2020;127(7):876–84.
78. Marchioni Beery RM, Vaziri H, Forouhar F. Primary biliary cirrhosis and primary sclerosing cholangitis: a review featuring a Women's health Perspective. J Clin Transl Hepatol 2014;2(4):266–84.

79. Efe C, Kahramanoğlu-Aksoy E, Yilmaz B, et al. Pregnancy in women with primary biliary cirrhosis. Autoimmun Rev 2014;13(9):931–5.

80. Poupon R, Chrétien Y, Chazouillères O, et al. Pregnancy in women with ursodeoxycholic acid-treated primary biliary cirrhosis. J Hepatol 2005;42(3):418–9.

81. Gossard AA, Lindor KD. Pregnancy in a patient with primary sclerosing cholangitis. J Clin Gastroenterol 2002;35(4):353–5.

82. Palmela C, Peerani F, Castaneda D, et al. Inflammatory bowel disease and primary sclerosing cholangitis: a review of the Phenotype and associated specific features. Gut Liver 2018;12(1):17–29.

83. Wellge BE, Sterneck M, Teufel A, et al. Pregnancy in primary sclerosing cholangitis. Gut 2011;60(8):1117–21.

84. Ludvigsson JF, Bergquist A, Ajne G, et al. A population-based cohort study of pregnancy outcomes among women with primary sclerosing cholangitis. Clin Gastroenterol Hepatol 2014;12(1):95–100.e1.

85. Chapman R, Fevery J, Kalloo A, et al. Diagnosis and management of primary sclerosing cholangitis. Hepatology 2010;51(2):660–78.

86. Tolunay HE, Aydın M, Cim N, et al. Maternal and fetal outcomes of pregnant women with hepatic cirrhosis. Gastroenterol Res Pract 2020;2020:5819819.

87. Stelmach A, Słowik Ł, Cichoń B, et al. Esophageal varices during pregnancy in the course of cirrhosis. Eur Rev Med Pharmacol Sci 2020;24(18):9615–7.

88. Zvárová V, Dolina J, Šenkyřík M, et al. Liver cirrhosis and pregnancy: a case report and review of literature. Vnitr Lek 2021;67(E-3):28–32. Jaterní cirhóza a těhotenství: kazuistika a přehled literatury.

89. Westbrook RH, Yeoman AD, O'Grady JG, et al. Model for end-stage liver disease score predicts outcome in cirrhotic patients during pregnancy. Clin Gastroenterol Hepatol 2011;9(8):694–9.

90. Shaheen AA, Myers RP. The outcomes of pregnancy in patients with cirrhosis: a population-based study. Liver Int 2010;30(2):275–83.

91. Savage C, Patel J, Lepe MR, et al. Transjugular intrahepatic portosystemic shunt creation for recurrent gastrointestinal bleeding during pregnancy. J Vasc Interv Radiol 2007;18(7):902–4.

92. Abbas MA, Stone WM, Fowl RJ, et al. Splenic artery aneurysms: two decades experience at Mayo clinic. Ann Vasc Surg 2002;16(4):442–9.

93. Rahim MN, Pirani T, Williamson C, et al. Management of pregnancy in women with cirrhosis. United Eur Gastroenterol J 2021;9(1):110–9.

94. Rasheed SM, Abdel Monem AM, Abd Ellah AH, et al. Prognosis and determinants of pregnancy outcome among patients with post-hepatitis liver cirrhosis. Int J Gynaecol Obstet 2013;121(3):247–51.

95. Wood AM, Grotegut CA, Ronald J, et al. Identification and management of abdominal Wall varices in pregnancy. Obstet Gynecol 2018;132(4):882–7.

96. Flemming JA, Mullin M, Lu J, et al. Outcomes of pregnant women with cirrhosis and their infants in a population-based study. Gastroenterology 2020;159(5):1752–62.e10.

97. Tan J, Surti B, Saab S. Pregnancy and cirrhosis. Liver Transpl 2008;14(8):1081–91.

Alcohol-Related Liver Disease Including New Developments

Parita Virendra Patel, MD[a], Steven L. Flamm, MD[b],*

KEYWORDS

• Alcohol use disorder • Alcohol-related liver disease • Early transplantation

KEY POINTS

- With the increasing rates of harmful alcohol use, screening for AUD and alcohol-related liver disease (ALD) is of the utmost importance.
- ALD is a spectrum of disease where continued, significant alcohol use can cause progression from fatty changes in the liver to inflammation, fibrosis, and eventually cirrhosis.
- Corticosteroids are the mainstay treatment of alcohol-associated hepatitis currently. However, potential novel therapies are under investigation.
- Early liver transplantation is an option for select patients with severe alcohol-associated hepatitis. Further studies evaluating the risks of post liver transplantation relapse are very much needed.

INTRODUCTION

The rate of alcohol consumption and prevalence of alcohol use disorder (AUD) is on the rise. In fact, 1 in 12 adults in the United States report heavy alcohol consumption, which is defined as 2 drinks per day for women and more than 3 drinks per day for men, or by participation in binge drinking (consumption of >5 drinks in men and >4 drinks in women over a span of 2 hours in one occasion).[1,2] Excessive alcohol use is the fifth leading risk factor for premature death and disability[3,4] and is associated with increased risk of accidents, increased medical and mental health costs, and increase in workplace productivity losses.[5] This high morbidity and mortality is due to the increasing rate of AUD, which is defined in the Diagnostic and Statistical Manual for Mental Disorders, fifth edition, as a pattern of alcohol consumption that results in at least 2 of the 11 listed criteria, with the severity of AUD defined by the number

a Piedmont Transplant Institute Liver Diseases and Transplantation, 1968 Peachtree Road Northwest, 77 Building 6th Floor, Atlanta, GA 30309, USA; b Department of Gastroenterology and Hepatology, Rush University Medical Center, 1620 West Harrison Street, Chicago, IL 60612, USA
* Corresponding author.
E-mail address: SFLAMM3@OUTLOOK.COM

Clin Liver Dis 27 (2023) 157–172
https://doi.org/10.1016/j.cld.2022.08.005
1089-3261/23/© 2022 Elsevier Inc. All rights reserved.

liver.theclinics.com

of criteria met[3,6] (**Table 1**). One-third of all adults in the United States will meet criteria for AUD at some point, whereas 15.1 million individuals will have met criteria for AUD in the past 12 months.[3,6]

Sustained, excessive alcohol use can eventually lead to inflammatory changes in the liver, resulting in alcoholic steatohepatitis (ASH) or alcohol-associated hepatitis (AH).[7] Although alcohol cessation can reverse hepatic steatosis and even fibrosis, cirrhosis cannot be reversed and can progress to episodes of decompensation and hepatocellular carcinoma (HCC) despite complete cessation of alcohol use.[1] Approximately, 10% to 20% of patients with alcohol-related liver disease (ALD) will develop cirrhosis, with the highest risk in patients with AH.[8] Mortality from alcohol-associated cirrhosis (AC) continues to increase, particularly in younger patients aged 25 to 34 years,[7,9] and accounts for 10% of all alcohol attributable deaths.[10] With this growing burden of disease, ALD is one of the leading indications for liver transplantation in the United States.[7] Understanding the diagnosis and treatment of both AUD and ALD is vital because the prevalence, mortality, and morbidity of these disorders continue to increase exponentially, and intervention can often ameliorate adverse outcomes.

Screening and Diagnosis Alcohol Use Disorder

As AUD and ALD are closely intertwined, it is essential to screen for and assess the level of alcohol use in patients before the development of ALD. Obtaining a detailed

Table 1 Diagnostic and statistical manual for mental disorders, fifth edition criteria for alcohol use disorder[69]	
In the Past Year, Have You:	
1.	Had times when you ended up drinking more, or longer, than you intended?
2.	More than once wanted to cut down or stop drinking, or tried to, but couldn't?
3.	Spent a lot of time drinking? Or being sick or getting over aftereffects?
4.	Wanted a drink so badly you couldn't think of anything else?
5.	Found that drinking – or being sick from drinking, often interfered with taking care of your home or family? Or caused job troubles? Or school problems?
6.	Continued to drink even though it was causing trouble with your family or friends?
7.	Given up or cut back on activities that were important or interesting to you, or gave you pleasure, in order to drink?
8.	More than once gotten into situations while or after drinking that increased your chances of getting hurt (such as driving, swimming, using machinery, walking in a dangerous area, or having unsafe sex)?
9.	Continued to drink even thought it was making you feel depressed or anxious or adding to another health problem? Or after having had a memory blackout?
10.	Had to drink much more than you once did to get the effect you want? Or found that your usual number of drinks had much less effect than before?
11.	Found that when the effects of alcohol were wearing off, you had withdrawal symptoms, such as trouble sleeping, shakiness, restlessness, nausea, sweating, a racing heart, or a seizure? Or sensed things that were not there?

Presence of at least 2 of these symptoms indicates AUD. The severity of AUD is defined as: Mild: presence of 2 to 3 symptoms. Moderate: presence of 4 to 5 symptoms. Severe: presence of 6 or more symptoms.

history on alcohol consumption can be difficult. Many patients may feel stigmatized or judged when asked about alcohol use, which can therefore lead to underreporting.[11] To minimize this risk, the American Association for the Study of Liver Disease (AASLD) recommends maintaining therapeutic alliance by creating a nonjudgmental, open and accepting interview style. Additionally, every opportunity, whether inpatient, outpatient, or in the emergency room (ER), should be used to screen for and identify patients with AUD.[7,12] The National Institute on Alcohol Abuse and Alcoholism recommends screening all patients by asking, "How many times in the past year have you had 5 or more drinks in a day (for men) or 4 or more drinks in a day (for women)."[13] Additional questions using the Alcohol Use Disorders Inventory Test (AUDIT) are then recommended for individuals who report even one episode of excessive drinking (**Table 2**). The AUDIT questionnaire is widely used and focuses on alcohol consumption patterns, dependence symptoms and any alcohol-associated problems.[7,14]

Although helpful in the prediction of harmful alcohol use, completion of AUDIT can be time-consuming for both patients and providers. As such, a shorter version called AUDIT-C has been validated as a more efficient method of screening for harmful alcohol use and performs better than the CAGE questionnaire.[15] In a prospective single site study, 141 patient's alcohol status was assessed by a hepatologist, an addiction specialist, and the AUDIT-C questionnaire. Alcohol consumption was identified by the hepatologist in 21.9% of patients, compared with 36.8% by the AUDIT-C questionnaire,[16] highlighting the clinical utility of such screening tools.

Treatment of Alcohol Use Disorder

Patients with scores concerning for harmful drinking (>8 on AUDIT, or $\geq$ 4 on AUDIT-C) should be referred for treatment.[7] Although screening and brief interventions can be effective for less severe alcohol misuse, it is unlikely to be helpful in patients with severe AUD. Additionally, given the high frequency of concomitant psychiatric comorbidities such as anxiety and depression in patients with AUD, referral to a mental health provider can be helpful. Treatment modalities include inpatient alcohol rehabilitation, group therapies, one-on-one therapies, family/couples counseling, and mutual aid societies. Determining which treatment modalities are best should be determined by an addiction specialist in conjunction with patient preference.[7] Relapse prevention pharmacotherapy should also be used concomitantly. Disulfiram, naltrexone, and acamprosate are all approved by the food and drug administration (FDA), whereas baclofen, gabapentin, and topiramate are additional considerations but not yet approved for AUD treatment.[7] Both behavioral and pharmacologic treatments are effective in decreasing risk of decompensation at 1 year (hazards ratio [HR] 0.85, $P < .001$) in patients with AC.[17]

Alcohol biomarkers, which are moieties in the blood, urine, or hair that can identify alcohol metabolites, can be helpful to aid diagnosis or support patients through recovery. Although there are no guidelines on how to best integrate biomarkers into AUD treatment, AASLD strongly recommends not to use these markers as a means to catch or punish patients and should be discussed with patients before testing.[7,12] Commonly used biomarkers include phosphatidylethanol (PEth), and urine ethyl glucuronide (EtG) and urine ethyl sulfate (EtS). PEth is a phospholipid with a half-life of 10 to 14 days but can be longer in patients with chronic, repeated episodes of heavy alcohol consumption. It is not influenced by body mass index, kidney, or liver disease but some studies have shown that women may have higher levels for a given amount of alcohol consumed when compared with men.[18] It can also provide additional information on the amount of alcohol consumed, with lower levels indicative of light or no drinking. In patients with chronic liver disease, PEth has been validated at a cutoff of

Table 2
Alcohol use disorders inventory test alcohol screening tool

	0	1	2	3	4
How often do you have a drink containing alcohol?	Never	Monthly or less	2–4 times a month	2–3 times a week	4+ times a week
How many drinks containing alcohol do you have on a typical day when you are drinking?	1–2	3 or 4	5 or 6	7–9	10 or more
How often do you have six or more standard drinks on one occasion?	Never	Less than monthly	Monthly	Weekly	Daily or almost daily
How often during the last year have you found that you were not able to stop drinking once you had started?	Never	Less than monthly	Monthly	Weekly	Daily or almost daily
How often during the last year have you failed to do what was normally expected of you because of drinking?	Never	Less than monthly	Monthly	Weekly	Daily or almost daily
How often during the last year have you needed a drink first thing in the morning to get yourself going after a heavy drinking session?	Never	Less than monthly	Monthly	Weekly	Daily or almost daily
How often during the last year have you had a feeling of guilty or remorse after drinking?	Never	Less than monthly	Monthly	Weekly	Daily or almost daily
How often during the last year have you been unable to remember what happened the night before because of your drinking?	Never	Less than monthly	Monthly	Weekly	Daily or almost daily
Have you or someone else been injured because of your drinking	No		Yes, but not in the last year		Yes, during the last year
Has a relative, friend, doctor or other healthcare worker been concerned about your drinking or suggested you cut down?	No		Yes, but not in the last year		Yes, during the last year

80 ng/mL for 4 drinks per day or more in recent weeks with a sensitivity of 91% and specificity of 77%.[19]

Less than 1% of alcohol is metabolized by uridine 5'-diphospho-glucuronosyltransferase and sulfotransferase, producing EtG and EtS. Although these are excreted in the urine, they can also be found in hair and blood. These can detect alcohol use up to 3 to 5 days before testing but detection times can be prolonged in renal failure.[12]

Carbohydrate-deficient transferring can also be used as a biomarker for chronic alcohol use. It is a measure of impaired transferrin glycosylation in the presence of alcohol and has a half-life of 2 to 3 weeks. Importantly, it can only detect alcohol if more than 60g is consumed. Cautious interpretation of results is advisable given an overall low sensitivity of 25% to 50% and false positives noted in patients with impaired liver function.[7,12,20,21] With the limitations of each biomarker, these tests should be used in conjunction with other laboratory data and clinical history to confirm or refute alcohol use.

Pathophysiology of Alcohol-Related Liver Disease

ALD is a spectrum of disease, and a long-term, significant alcohol use can lead to progression from hepatic steatosis to steatohepatitis, fibrosis, and eventually cirrhosis. Risk factors associated with increased risk of ALD include alcohol ingestion of more than 1 drink/d for women, 2 drinks/d for men, binge drinking or drinking while fasting, smoking cigarettes, female gender, and increased BMI. Genetic variants including PNPLA3 and TM6SF2 have been associated with an increased risk of AC and AH.[22] Finally, in patients with concomitant liver disease, particularly nonalcoholic fatty liver disease (NAFLD), hepatitis C virus (HCV), and hemochromatosis, the risk of developing advanced fibrosis and cirrhosis is markedly increased, even with moderate use of alcohol. In a nationwide retrospective study in France of more than 90,000 HCV patients, patients with AUD had the highest odds for liver-related complications, more than two-thirds of liver transplantation, and more than 60,000 liver-related deaths.[23] Another study of 224 patients with hemochromatosis found that those who drank more than 60g of alcohol per day were 9 times more likely to develop cirrhosis than those who drank less than this amount.[24]

Pathogenesis of ALD is multifactorial and has been linked to ethanol-mediated liver injury, inflammatory immune response to injury and intestinal permeability and microbiome changes.[25] Steatosis, which is the initial insult noted in patients with heavy alcohol use, is due to accumulation of triglycerides, phospholipids, and cholesterol esters in hepatocytes via numerous transcription factors involved in fatty acid synthesis and oxidation.[26]

Additionally, acetaldehyde (AA), the first metabolite of alcohol degradation, is one of the main contributors to the development of ALD.[26] AA has been shown to be highly reactive and mutagenic, and linked to alcohol-related toxicity, and ultimately hepatocyte death. Damaged hepatocytes release endogenous damage-associated molecular patterns, which then can activate cellular pattern recognition receptors, ultimately results in inflammation.[25]

Alcohol ingestion can also increase gut permeability and facilitate the translocation of bacterial endotoxins such as lipopolysaccharides into portal blood. Once these endotoxins reach the Kupffer cells, proinflammatory cascades are activated and contribute to hepatocellular damage.[26]

Diagnosis of Alcohol-Related Liver Disease

As the initial stages of ALD can be asymptomatic or present with nonspecific findings, making an early clinical diagnosis of ALD can be challenging. As such, patients with significant alcohol use should be screened for ALD with serum liver chemistries and ultrasonography. Typically, elevation in liver enzymes secondary to alcohol use are not more than 5 times the upper limit of normal, and present with AST 2 or 3 times greater than ALT in the setting of AH.[27,28] Discriminant indices, such as the ALD/NAFLD index (ANI) can help differentiate between nonalcoholic fatty liver disease and ALD.

Hepatic Steatosis

Hepatic steatosis is asymptomatic in most patients. Elevated aspartate transaminase (AST) and gamma-glutamyl transferase (GGT) can be helpful markers of recent alcohol consumption. Typically, steatosis is found incidentally on imaging modalities, and liver biopsy is generally unnecessary for diagnosis. MRI is the most accurate modality in quantification of fat content over the entire volume of the liver.[7,29] Ultrasonography, however, is cheaper and more easily obtainable, and can detect moderate-to-severe steatosis with a sensitivity and specificity of 90%.[27,30]

Alcohol-Associated Cirrhosis

Similarly, most patients with compensated AC remain asymptomatic. Thrombocytopenia as a result of splenic sequestration of platelets from portal hypertension is often present but other laboratory values may be normal. Patients can be assessed for cirrhosis using modalities such as the FibroTest, which uses blood serum markers to generate a score that can then be correlated to the degree of fibrosis present. Additionally, radiologic modalities such as transient elastography and magnetic resonance elastography can provide an estimate of liver stiffness. It is important to diagnosis cirrhosis even if asymptomatic because patients with cirrhosis have increased the risk of HCC and should be screened with semiannual liver imaging.

Elevated bilirubin, prothrombin time, and decreased albumin can be helpful and suggest more advanced ALD. However, cirrhosis is often diagnosed during episodes of decompensation with ascites, hepatic encephalopathy, jaundice, or gastrointestinal bleeding related to varices.[7,27] The prognosis is much worse in the setting of decompensated disease.

Alcohol-Associated Hepatitis

Patients with AH typically present with jaundice, serum bilirubin levels greater than 3 mg/dL, elevated serum aminotransferase levels with an elevated ratio of AST to alanine transaminase (ALT), and have a clinical history of at least one alcoholic drink within 8 weeks of jaundice onset. Patients with AH can present with a broad spectrum of symptoms ranging from jaundice to liver failure. In certain cases where the diagnosis remains elusive, a liver biopsy may be needed but this is typically not required. Underlying cirrhosis can be difficult to distinguish in patients with acute AH. Fibrosis is often overestimated by noninvasive methods during an acute AH episode (particularly elastography), and therefore should not be assessed for at least 6 months after alcohol cessation.

Prognostic Scoring

Several serum-based scoring systemics have been evaluated for predicting outcomes and classifying severity of ALD. Although clinical features such as ascites and jaundice can be helpful, laboratory markers are more useful and accurate in predicting outcomes in patients with AH.[31] The Maddrey discriminant function, which was first published in 1978, has been the most commonly used model to identify the optimal candidates for corticosteroid therapy. Short-term mortality for patients with maddrey discriminant function (DF) less than 32, or nonsevere disease, is 10%, compared with 30% to 60% for those with DF greater than 32, or severe disease. Therefore, corticosteroids are typically started in patients with DF greater than 32 because they likely have the greatest potential benefit from treatment.[32,33]

The Lille score is used to assess response to corticosteroid treatment, by calculating a score based on age, albumin, prothrombin time (PT), and bilirubin on day 0 and day 7. A Lille score less than 0.45 has been associated with 15% mortality at 6 months compared with 75% mortality for patients with a score of 0.45 of greater. As such, patients with a score of 0.45 or greater on day 7 of treatment indicate a lack of response to corticosteroids and should be used to guide cessation of treatment.[34,35] Further studies have shown that the use of the Lille score at day 4 is just as accurate as day 7 in predicting response to corticosteroids and can be used at an earlier time point to discontinue therapy.[36]

Although not used to guide treatment, the age, bilirubin, INR, creatinine score, allows stratification of risk of death in patients with AH at 90 days and 1 year. Low-risk patients with scores less than 6.71 are associated with a 90-day mortality of 0% compared with 75% in high-risk patients with score greater than 9.0.[37] Similarly, the model for end stage liver disease (MELD) score has been evaluated in a retrospective study to predict mortality. In fact, a MELD score greater than 20 had a sensitivity and specificity of 0.75 in predicting 90-day mortality in patients with AH.[38]

Current Treatment of Alcohol-Associated Hepatitis

Continued alcohol abstinence has been shown to reduce the risk of decompensating events including variceal bleeding, ascites, hepatic encephalopathy, and the risk of developing HCC.[39–41] In a study of 398 patients, there was a dose effect of alcohol on the hazard ratio of death: 2.36 (P = .052) for 1 to 29 g/d, 3.2 (P = .003) for 30 to 49 g/d, and 3.51 (P < .0001) for 50 to 99 g/d and 5.61 (P < .0001) for 100 g or greater per day.[42,43] In another study of 142 patients with AH, complete abstinence was associated with better long-term survival (HR 0.53, P = .03). Therefore, complete alcohol cessation should be strongly recommended to all patients with ALD.

Given the close interplay between ALD and AUD, both the AASLD and European Association for the Study of Liver recommend integration of a multidisciplinary care team as a method of effective treatment. Although hepatology and gastroenterology providers screen for AUD, recent surveys found that 71% never prescribed AUD pharmacotherapy due to low comfort levels.[44] As a result, creating more collaborative AUD and ALD treatment models can allow patients to receive the full range of beneficial treatment of both disorders.[12]

Pharmacologic Therapy

Corticosteroids have been the most extensively studied treatment of AH with several clinical trials performed during the past 40 years. Most notably, the STOPAH trial randomized 1103 patients with severe AH between 2011 and 2014 to receive prednisolone 40 mg/d, pentoxifylline (PTX) 400 mg 3 times a day, combination of PTX and prednisolone, or placebo. The study did not find a statistically significant survival benefit at 28 days in patients receiving prednisolone compared with those who received placebo. On a post hoc multivariate analysis, corticosteroids were found to have a survival benefit at 28 days (odds ratio [OR] 0.61, P = .015) but not at 90 days or 1 year.

Further studies with concomitant corticosteroids and n-acetylcysteine (NAC) treatment demonstrated lower mortality at 1 month (8% vs 24%, P = .006), and decreased rate of death due to hepatorenal syndrome (9% vs 22%, P = .02). At 3 and 6 months, however, no significant difference in mortality was observed (22% vs 34%, $P = .06$).[45] In a meta-analysis of 22 randomized controlled trials, short-term morality reduction was noted with the addition of NAC to corticosteroids.[46] Therefore, the combination of NAC and corticosteroids still warrants further investigation, and although it can be considered in the treatment of patients with AH, it is not yet recommended.[7]

In patients with severe AH, beta-blockers have been associated with worsening renal function. In a retrospective study of 139 patients of which 48 received noncardio-selective beta-blocker, there was no difference in transplantation free mortality at 6 months ($P = .25$) but the incidence of acute renal injury was higher in patients who received a beta-blocker (89.6% vs 50.4%, $P = .0001$).[47] Beta-blockers in patients with severe AH should only be used with great caution.

Nutritional Therapy

Malnutrition is commonly observed in patients with ALD, with more severe malnutrition associated with higher mortality and morbidity.[33] Reduced oral intake, amount, and duration of alcohol use, slowed gut motility, and malabsorption are all possible factors that contribute to malnutrition in patients with AH.[33] Those who are unable to meet caloric requirements should be offered oral protein supplements, and those who are unable to swallow should be provided nasogastric or nasojejunal feeding. Parenteral nutrition is recommended for those who are unable to receive oral nutritional or enteral nutrition supplementation.[33] In a randomized controlled trial of ICU patients with severe AH, a greater proportion of patients who consumed less than 21.5 kcal/kg/d died (65.8%, 95%CI 48.8–78.4) compared with patients with higher caloric intake (33.1% 95%CI 23.1%-43.4%, $P < .001$).[48]

Folate, thiamine, pyridoxine, vitamins A, B12, D, and E, and zinc are commonly deficient due to poor oral intake and malabsorption in patients with advanced ALD. Thiamine supplementation is key to preventing Wernicke encephalopathy and Korsakoff psychosis. Zinc supplementation has also been shown to improve clinical outcomes, and attenuates hepatic inflammation and steatosis, improve insulin resistance, and improve the grade of HE.[33,49]

Novel Treatment Agents

As the pathophysiology of AH is evolving, there is increasing interest in novel therapeutic agents (Table 3). One group of potential therapeutics is targeted against the inflammatory pathways that are thought to play a role in the pathogenesis of AH. Studies have shown that interleukin-1β (IL-1) is a central player in the pathogenesis of ALD and administration of IL-1 receptor antagonists can attenuate inflammation-dependent ASH in mice.[50,51] A randomized control trial involving Anakinra, a recombinant IL-1 receptor antagonist, for 14 days, zinc supplementation (to improve gut barrier function) for 180 days, and PTX (to decrease the risk of hepatorenal syndrome [HRS]) for 28 days resulted in similar survival at 28 days and a 22% better survival at 90 days and 190 days compared with patients treated with methylprednisolone, although the difference did not achieve statistical significance.[52] Treatment with canakinumab, a recombinant human monoclonal antibody against IL-1β, is currently under investigation, to evaluate histologic improvement after 28 days in patients with MELD less than 27 (NCT03775109).[51] Additionally, other inflammatory processes implicated in AH include caspase-dependent activation of inflammasomes and apoptosis triggered by alcohol use.[51] A placebo-controlled, multicenter, double-blind randomized clinical trial of emricasan was studied in patients with AH. However, due to high levels that exceeded levels in toxicology studies and a lack of reliable safe dosing, the trial was terminated after recruiting 5 patients (NCT01912404).[51]

Table 3
Novel therapies in alcohol associated hepatitis

Mode of Therapy	Therapeutic Agent	Mechanism of Action	Completed and/or Ongoing Clinical Trials
Inflammatory pathway		Alcohol can damage hepatocytes and result in the release of danger-associated molecular patterns which can lead to inflammatory responses in the liver	
	Anakinra	Recombinant IL-1 antagonist	NCT01809132
	Canakinumab	Recombinant human monoclonal antibody against IL-1β	NCT03775109
	Emricasan	Pan-caspase inhibitor	NCT01912404
Gut Liver Axis		Alcohol can lead to bacterial overgrowth, causing changes in the intestinal microbiome. Additional impairments in gut permeability leads to bacterial translocation and higher levels of bacterial products in the systemic circulation	
	Antibiotics	Intestinal decontamination	NCT03157388
	Probiotics	Restoration of bowel flora	NCT02335632
	Bovine colostrum	contains immuno- globulin G antibodies against lipopolysaccharide	NCT02473341
	Zinc	Regulates tight junctions between intestinal epithelial cells and controls bacterial translocation	NCT04072822
	Fecal microbiota transplant	Restore healthy intestinal flora	NCT02458079
Reducing oxidative stress		Production of reactive oxygen species increases cellular damage	
	NAC	Antioxidant that can restore glutathione, the main protective agent against oxidative stress in hepatocytes	NCT03069300
	Metadoxine	Antioxidant drug that reduces free fatty acid accumulation and inhibits tumor necrosis factor-α secretion	
Liver regeneration	G-CSF	Facilitates the mobilization of immune cells from bone marrow that may aid liver regeneration	NCT02442180, NCT03703674, NCT04066179
	IL-22	Displays anti-apoptotic, anti-oxidative, anti-lipogenic and proliferative effects in hepatocytes, and promotes the production of antimicrobial proteins	NCT02655510
	OCA	Selective farnesoid X agonist regulating bile acid synthesis and transport, reduces oxidative stress and portal hypertension. OCA also modulates carbohydrate and lipid metabolism and plays a role in liver regeneration after injury	NCT02039219

Modified from Tornai D, Szabo G. Emerging medical therapies for severe alcoholic hepatitis. Clin Mol Hepatol. 10 2020;26(4):686-696.

Agents targeting the gut–liver axis and modifying the microbiome are also under investigation. Alcohol consumption can lead to bacterial overgrowth, causing changes in the intestinal microbiome. Additional impairments in gut permeability lead to bacterial translocation and higher levels of bacterial products in the systemic circulation. Attempts at intestinal decontamination using rifaximin, vancomycin, bovine colostrum, and zinc supplementation have been studied or are under investigation.[51] Targeting the microbiome with probiotics has also been evaluated. In a small study of patients with mild–moderate AH, use of *Bifidobacterium bifidum* and *Lactobacillus plantarum* 8PA3 was associated with restoration of bowel flora and greater improvement in levels of AST, ALT, GGT, lactate dehydrogenase, and serum bilirubin compared with standard therapy for alcohol abstinence plus vitamins.[53] *Lactobacillus rhamnosus* has also been examined in a mouse model and may reduce endotoxemia and promote intestinal epithelial integrity.[54] *Lactobacillus* has been shown to inhibit activation of toll-like receptor and tumor necrosis factor-alpha production and thereby reduce alcohol-induced hepatic inflammation and injury in a study of mice receiving 8 weeks of alcohol feeding.[55] Fecal microbiota transplant (FMT), which has been studied in refractory C. Difficile infection, may also provide benefit in AH. In an open-label pilot study with 8 patients with corticosteroid refractory resistant AH, FMT from healthy donors was associated with reduced pathogen levels, increased levels of beneficial bacterial strains 1 year after treatment, and improved survival.[56] Several other trials are under investigation but many concerns persist given the potential of high-risk infections with this treatment.[31]

Agents aimed at stimulating hepatic regenerative properties are also under examination. Twenty-four patients with alcohol-related cirrhosis and concomitant alcohol-related steatohepatitis were randomized to 5 days of granulocyte colony stimulating factor (G-CSF) versus standard of care. In patients who received G-CSF, increases in the number of CD34+ cells and levels of hepatocyte growth factor and hepatic progenitor cells were observed, suggesting that G-CSF may stimulate liver regeneration in patients with AH.[31,57] In an open label single center study in India, 57 patients with severe AH were randomly assigned to groups that received standard medical therapy (with PTX) plus G-CSF for 5 days (G-CSF group; n = 18), standard medical therapy plus G-CSF and intravenous NAC for 5 days (combination group; n = 19), or standard medical therapy alone. A 90-day survival was higher in patients who received G-CSF with PTX or IV NAC compared with standard therapy alone.[58] Furthermore, IL-22 upregulates markers of regeneration while downregulating markers of inflammation in patients with AH.[59] Obeticholic acid (OCA), a farnesoid X receptor agonist, reduces oxidative stress and portal hypertension but also modulates carbohydrate and lipid metabolism, and plays a role in liver regeneration after injury. A phase 2, placebo-controlled, randomized trial aimed to test the effectiveness of OCA in patients with moderately severe AH. However, this was terminated after enrollment of 19 patients due to postmarketing reports of hepatotoxicity, primarily in patients with portal hypertension and/or decompensated disease (NCT02039219). In fact, a box warning has been issued to lower the dose of OCA from daily to weekly in patients with Child Pugh class B/C or with prior hepatic decompensation.[51]

Oxidative stress plays an important role in the pathogenesis of AH and is a focus of investigational therapies. Increased levels of reactive oxygen species are associated with reduced levels of glutathione, a protective agent against oxidative stress in hepatocytes.[51] NAC can restore glutathione but has not demonstrated survival benefit in AH patients when used alone.[60] Metadoxine can also increase the level of glutathione in hepatocytes and may reduce steatosis in animals fed with alcohol.[61] In a randomized open label clinical trial in Mexico, 70 patients with severe AH received either prednisone versus prednisone plus 500 mg of metadoxine 3 times a day. Addition of metadoxine to corticosteroid therapy improved survival at 30 days and 90 days and was associated with lower rates of encephalopathy and hepatorenal syndrome.[62]

Liver Transplantation

At a consensus conference of the AASLD and American Society of Transplantation in 1997, the 6-month alcohol abstinence rule before liver transplantation was created because experts thought this provided ample time to evaluate potential liver recovery from AH, as well as a patient's commitment to abstinence. As such, 85% of liver transplantation programs and 43% of third party payors in the United States required 6 months of abstinence before evaluation for a liver transplantation.[63–65] During the last several years, however, several studies have shown that adherence to the 6-month abstinence rule did not reliably predict relapse after transplantation.[64,66] Furthermore, the 6-month abstinence rule placed patients at a severe disadvantage because the short-term mortality for patients with corticosteroid refractory, severe AH was as high as 70%.[35] Given this bleak prognosis, early liver transplantation (before 6 months abstinence) was studied in patients with severe ALD. Seven centers in France and Belgium enrolled patients who met strict criteria to be considered for liver transplantation: no prior episodes of AH, Lille scores of 0.45 or higher, supportive family members, no severe coexisting conditions, and a commitment to alcohol abstinence. The cumulative 6-month survival rate was higher among patients who received early liver transplantation compared with those who did not ($P < .001$), with a benefit of early liver transplantation maintained through 2 years of follow-up ($P = .004$).[67] The American Consortium of Early Liver Transplantation confirmed these findings in a retrospective study consisting of 147 patients from 12 centers in 8 United Network for Organ Sharing regions. Among patients with severe AH and no previous diagnosis of liver disease who underwent liver transplantation before 6 months of abstinence, the cumulative patient survival percentages after liver transplantation (LT) were 94% at 1 year (95% CI 89%–97%) and 84% at 3 years (95% CI 75%–90%). The cumulative incidence of sustained alcohol use was 10% at 1 year (95% CI 6%–18%) and 17% at 3 years (95% CI 10%–27%) after LT.[68] Although great strides have been made in understanding the role of liver transplantation in severe AH, more studies are needed to understand how to best predict the risk of alcohol relapse after LT. Prediction models including Stanford Integrated Psychosocial Assessment for Transplantation, Alcohol Relapse Risk Assessment, and the Sustained Alcohol Use Post LT score have been proposed. However, given the complexity of AUD, it is unlikely for one single score to reliably predict the risk of relapse posttransplantation. As such, it is essential to approach both pretransplantation and posttransplantation care with a multidisciplinary approach.

SUMMARY

As the prevalence of AUD and ALD increases, it is of upmost importance to understand the best modalities of screening, diagnosis, and treatment of these disorders. Although early screening for ALD and early implementation of behavioral therapies is key, many strides have been made with medical therapeutics. Although corticosteroids remain the mainstay of treatment of severe AH at this time, the benefit is limited to a selected population. As such, several promising novel therapies for AH are under investigation, including drugs targeting inflammatory pathways, regenerative properties, and the gut–liver axis. During the last several years, early liver transplantation has also proven to be an effective treatment option in AH for a select patient population. However, optimal identification of patients at high risk of alcohol relapse is key to ensure ongoing success of liver transplantation in this population.

CLINICS CARE POINTS

- It is essential to screen for and assess the level of alcohol us in patients before the development of alcohol-related liver disease. Both Alcohol Use Disorders Inventory Test (AUDIT) and AUDIT-C have been validated as a screening tool for harmful alcohol use.
- Patients with scores greater than 8 on AUDIT or 4 or greater on AUDIT-C should be referred for treatment.
- Although underutilized, relapse prevention pharmacotherapy can be helpful. Disulfiram, naltrexone, and acamprosate are all approved by the FDA.
- Alcohol biomarkers, which are moieties in the blood, urine, or hair that can identify alcohol metabolites, can be helpful to aid diagnosis or support patients through recovery.
- Society guidelines recommend integration of a multidisciplinary care team as a method of effective treatment.
- Corticosteroids are the mainstay of treatment of alcohol-associated hepatitis currently but use is overall limited.
- Several novel agents targeting different pathways are under investigation.
- Early liver transplantation has proven to be effective in a very select population of patients with AH but ongoing studies in predicting posttransplant alcohol relapse are still needed.

DISCLOSURE

S.T. Flamm: Research with DURECT; P.V. Patel: no disclosures.

REFERENCES

1. Axley PD, Richardson CT, Singal AK. Epidemiology of alcohol consumption and societal burden of alcoholism and alcoholic liver disease. Clin Liver Dis 2019; 23(1):39–50.
2. Rehm J, Gmel GE, Gmel G, et al. The relationship between different dimensions of alcohol use and the burden of disease-an update. Addict 2017;112(6): 968–1001.
3. Witkiewitz K, Litten RZ, Leggio L. Advances in the science and treatment of alcohol use disorder. Sci Adv 2019;5(9):eaax4043.
4. Sacks JJ, Gonzales KR, Bouchery EE, et al. 2010 National and state costs of excessive alcohol consumption. Am J Prev Med 2015;49(5):e73–9.
5. Organization WH. Global Status Report on Alcohol and Health 2018. 2018. Available at: https://www.who.int/publications/i/item/9789241565639.
6. Grant BF, Goldstein RB, Saha TD, et al. Epidemiology of DSM-5 alcohol use disorder: results from the national epidemiologic survey on alcohol and related conditions III. JAMA Psychiatry 2015;72(8):757–66.
7. Crabb DW, Im GY, Szabo G, et al. Diagnosis and treatment of alcohol-associated liver diseases: 2019 practice guidance from the American association for the study of liver diseases. Hepatol 2020;71(1):306–33.
8. Gao B, Bataller R. Alcoholic liver disease: pathogenesis and new therapeutic targets. Gastroenterol 2011;141(5):1572–85.

9. Tapper EB, Parikh ND. Mortality due to cirrhosis and liver cancer in the United States, 1999-2016: observational study. BMJ 2018;362:k2817.

10. Rehm J, Shield KD. Global burden of alcohol use disorders and alcohol liver disease. Biomedicines 2019;7(4). https://doi.org/10.3390/biomedicines7040099.

11. Vaughn-Sandler V, Sherman C, Aronsohn A, et al. Consequences of perceived stigma among patients with cirrhosis. Dig Dis Sci 2014;59(3):681–6.

12. Mellinger JL, Winder GS. Alcohol use disorders in alcoholic liver disease. Clin Liver Dis 2019;23(1):55–69.

13. Smith PC, Schmidt SM, Allensworth-Davies D, et al. Primary care validation of a single-question alcohol screening test. J Gen Intern Med 2009;24(7):783–8.

14. Saunders JB, Aasland OG, Babor TF, et al. Development of the alcohol use disorders identification test (AUDIT): WHO collaborative project on early detection of persons with harmful alcohol consumption–II. Addict 1993;88(6):791–804.

15. Bradley KA, DeBenedetti AF, Volk RJ, et al. AUDIT-C as a brief screen for alcohol misuse in primary care. Alcohol Clin Exp Res 2007;31(7):1208–17.

16. Donnadieu-Rigole H, Olive L, Nalpas B, et al. Follow-up of alcohol consumption after liver transplantation: interest of an addiction team? Alcohol Clin Exp Res 2017;41(1):165–70.

17. Mellinger JL, Fernandez A, Shedden K, et al. Gender Disparities in alcohol use disorder treatment among privately insured patients with alcohol-associated cirrhosis. Alcohol Clin Exp Res 2019;43(2):334–41.

18. Simon TW. Providing context for phosphatidylethanol as a biomarker of alcohol consumption with a pharmacokinetic model. Regul Toxicol Pharmacol 2018;94:163–71.

19. Stewart SH, Koch DG, Willner IR, et al. Validation of blood phosphatidylethanol as an alcohol consumption biomarker in patients with chronic liver disease. Alcohol Clin Exp Res 2014;38(6):1706–11.

20. Berlakovich GA, Soliman T, Freundorfer E, et al. Pretransplant screening of sobriety with carbohydrate-deficient transferrin in patients suffering from alcoholic cirrhosis. Transpl Int 2004;17(10):617–21.

21. DiMartini A, Day N, Lane T, et al. Carbohydrate deficient transferrin in abstaining patients with end-stage liver disease. Alcohol Clin Exp Res 2001;25(12):1729–33.

22. Stickel F, Moreno C, Hampe J, et al. The genetics of alcohol dependence and alcohol-related liver disease. J Hepatol 2017;66(1):195–211.

23. Schwarzinger M, Baillot S, Yazdanpanah Y, et al. Contribution of alcohol use disorders on the burden of chronic hepatitis C in France, 2008-2013: a nationwide retrospective cohort study. J Hepatol 2017;67(3):454–61.

24. Fletcher LM, Dixon JL, Purdie DM, et al. Excess alcohol greatly increases the prevalence of cirrhosis in hereditary hemochromatosis. Gastroenterology 2002;122(2):281–9.

25. Dunn W, Shah VH. Pathogenesis of alcoholic liver disease. Clin Liver Dis 2016;20(3):445–56.

26. Stickel F, Datz C, Hampe J, et al. Pathophysiology and management of alcoholic liver disease: update 2016. Gut Liver 2017;11(2):173–88.

27. Singal AK, Mathurin P. Diagnosis and treatment of alcohol-associated liver disease: a review. JAMA 2021;326(2):165–76.

28. Sharma P, Arora A. Clinical presentation of alcoholic liver disease and non-alcoholic fatty liver disease: spectrum and diagnosis. Transl Gastroenterol Hepatol 2020;5:19.

29. Reeder SB, Cruite I, Hamilton G, et al. Quantitative assessment of liver fat with magnetic resonance imaging and spectroscopy. J Magn Reson Imaging 2011; 34(4):729–49.

30. Hernaez R, Lazo M, Bonekamp S, et al. Diagnostic accuracy and reliability of ultrasonography for the detection of fatty liver: a meta-analysis. Hepatology 2011; 54(3):1082–90.

31. Mitchell MC, Kerr T, Herlong HF. Current management and future treatment of alcoholic hepatitis. Gastroenterol Hepatol (N Y) 2020;16(4):178–89.

32. Carithers RL, Herlong HF, Diehl AM, et al. Methylprednisolone therapy in patients with severe alcoholic hepatitis. A randomized multicenter trial. Ann Intern Med 1989;110(9):685–90.

33. Siddiqi FA, Sajja KC, Latt NL. Current management of alcohol-associated liver disease. Gastroenterol Hepatol (N Y) 2020;16(11):561–70.

34. Hosseini N, Shor J, Szabo G. Alcoholic hepatitis: a review. Alcohol Alcohol 2019; 54(4):408–16.

35. Louvet A, Naveau S, Abdelnour M, et al. The Lille model: a new tool for therapeutic strategy in patients with severe alcoholic hepatitis treated with steroids. *Hepatol* Jun 2007;45(6):1348–54.

36. Garcia-Saenz-de-Sicilia M, Duvoor C, Altamirano J, et al. A day-4 Lille model predicts response to corticosteroids and mortality in severe alcoholic hepatitis. Am J Gastroenterol 2017;112(2):306–15.

37. Dominguez M, Rincón D, Abraldes JG, et al. A new scoring system for prognostic stratification of patients with alcoholic hepatitis. Am J Gastroenterol 2008;103(11): 2747–56.

38. Dunn W, Jamil LH, Brown LS, et al. MELD accurately predicts mortality in patients with alcoholic hepatitis. Hepatol 2005;41(2):353–8.

39. Lucey MR, Connor JT, Boyer TD, et al. Alcohol consumption by cirrhotic subjects: patterns of use and effects on liver function. Am J Gastroenterol 2008;103(7): 1698–706.

40. Verrill C, Markham H, Templeton A, et al. Alcohol-related cirrhosis–early abstinence is a key factor in prognosis, even in the most severe cases. Addiction 2009;104(5):768–74.

41. Potts JR, Goubet S, Heneghan MA, et al. Determinants of long-term outcome in severe alcoholic hepatitis. Aliment Pharmacol Ther 2013;38(6):584–95.

42. Louvet A, Labreuche J, Artru F, et al. Main drivers of outcome differ between short term and long term in severe alcoholic hepatitis: a prospective study. Hepatology 2017;66(5):1464–73.

43. Altamirano J, López-Pelayo H, Michelena J, et al. Alcohol abstinence in patients surviving an episode of alcoholic hepatitis: prediction and impact on long-term survival. Hepatology 2017;66(6):1842–53.

44. Im GY, Mellinger JL, Winters A, et al. Provider attitudes and practices for alcohol screening, treatment, and education in patients with liver disease: a survey from the American association for the study of liver diseases alcohol-associated liver disease special interest group. Clin Gastroenterol Hepatol 2021;19(11): 2407–16.e8.

45. Nguyen-Khac E, Thevenot T, Piquet MA, et al. Glucocorticoids plus N-acetylcysteine in severe alcoholic hepatitis. N Engl J Med 2011;365(19):1781–9.

46. Singh S, Murad MH, Chandar AK, et al. Comparative effectiveness of pharmacological interventions for severe alcoholic hepatitis: a systematic review and Network meta-analysis. Gastroenterology 2015;149(4):958–70.e12.

47. Sersté T, Njimi H, Degré D, et al. The use of beta-blockers is associated with the occurrence of acute kidney injury in severe alcoholic hepatitis. Liver Int 2015; 35(8):1974–82.

48. Moreno C, Deltenre P, Senterre C, et al. Intensive enteral nutrition is ineffective for patients with severe alcoholic hepatitis treated with corticosteroids. *Gastroenterol* Apr 2016;150(4):903–10.e8.

49. Himoto T, Masaki T. Associations between zinc deficiency and metabolic abnormalities in patients with chronic liver disease. Nutrients 2018;10(1). https://doi.org/10.3390/nu10010088.

50. Petrasek J, Bala S, Csak T, et al. IL-1 receptor antagonist ameliorates inflammasome-dependent alcoholic steatohepatitis in mice. J Clin Invest 2012; 122(10):3476–89.

51. Tornai D, Szabo G. Emerging medical therapies for severe alcoholic hepatitis. Clin Mol Hepatol 2020;26(4):686–96.

52. Szabo G, Mitchell M, McClain CJ, et al. IL-1 receptor antagonist plus pentoxifylline and zinc for severe alcohol-associated hepatitis. Hepatol 2022;27. https://doi.org/10.1002/hep.32478.

53. Kirpich IA, Solovieva NV, Leikhter SN, et al. Probiotics restore bowel flora and improve liver enzymes in human alcohol-induced liver injury: a pilot study. Alcohol 2008;42(8):675–82.

54. Wang Y, Liu Y, Sidhu A, et al. Lactobacillus rhamnosus GG culture supernatant ameliorates acute alcohol-induced intestinal permeability and liver injury. Am J Physiol Gastrointest Liver Physiol 2012;303(1):G32–41.

55. Wang Y, Liu Y, Kirpich I, et al. Lactobacillus rhamnosus GG reduces hepatic TNFα production and inflammation in chronic alcohol-induced liver injury. *J Nutr Biochem* Sep 2013;24(9):1609–15.

56. Philips CA, Pande A, Shasthry SM, et al. Healthy donor fecal microbiota transplantation in steroid-ineligible severe alcoholic hepatitis: a pilot study. Clin Gastroenterol Hepatol 2017;15(4):600–2.

57. Spahr L, Lambert JF, Rubbia-Brandt L, et al. Granulocyte-colony stimulating factor induces proliferation of hepatic progenitors in alcoholic steatohepatitis: a randomized trial. Hepatology 2008;48(1):221–9.

58. Singh V, Keisham A, Bhalla A, et al. Efficacy of granulocyte colony-stimulating factor and N-acetylcysteine therapies in patients with severe alcoholic hepatitis. Clin Gastroenterol Hepatol 2018;16(10):1650–6.e2.

59. Arab JP, Sehrawat TS, Simonetto DA, et al. An open-label, dose-escalation study to assess the safety and efficacy of IL-22 agonist F-652 in patients with alcohol-associated hepatitis. Hepatol 2020;72(2):441–53.

60. Stewart S, Prince M, Bassendine M, et al. A randomized trial of antioxidant therapy alone or with corticosteroids in acute alcoholic hepatitis. J Hepatol 2007; 47(2):277–83.

61. Calabrese V, Calderone A, Ragusa N, et al. Effects of Metadoxine on cellular status of glutathione and of enzymatic defence system following acute ethanol intoxication in rats. Drugs Exp Clin Res 1996;22(1):17–24.

62. Higuera-de la Tijera F, Servín-Caamaño AI, Cruz-Herrera J, et al. Treatment with metadoxine and its impact on early mortality in patients with severe alcoholic hepatitis. Ann Hepatol 2014;13(3):343–52.

63. Weinrieb RM, Van Horn DH, McLellan AT, et al. Interpreting the significance of drinking by alcohol-dependent liver transplant patients: fostering candor is the key to recovery. Liver Transpl 2000;6(6):769–76.

64. Leong J, Im GY. Evaluation and selection of the patient with alcoholic liver disease for liver transplant. Clin Liver Dis 2012;16(4):851–63.

65. Everhart JE, Beresford TP. Liver transplantation for alcoholic liver disease: a survey of transplantation programs in the United States. Liver Transpl Surg 1997; 3(3):220–6.

66. Yates WR, Martin M, LaBrecque D, et al. A model to examine the validity of the 6-month abstinence criterion for liver transplantation. Alcohol Clin Exp Res 1998; 22(2):513–7.

67. Mathurin P, Moreno C, Samuel D, et al. Early liver transplantation for severe alcoholic hepatitis. N Engl J Med 2011;365(19):1790–800.

68. Lee BP, Mehta N, Platt L, et al. Outcomes of early liver transplantation for patients with severe alcoholic hepatitis. Gastroenterology 2018;155(2):422–30.e1.

69. Hasin DS, O'Brien CP, Auriacombe M, et al. DSM-5 criteria for substance use disorders: recommendations and rationale. Am J Psychiatry 2013;170(8):834–51.

Printed and bound by CPI Group (UK) Ltd, Croydon, CR0 4YY

03/10/2024

01040467-0014